Unhealthy Societies

Among the developed countries it is not the richest societies which have the best health, but those that have the smallest income differences between rich and poor. Inequality and relative poverty have absolute effects: they increase death rates. But why? How can smaller income differences raise average life expectancy?

Using examples from the USA, Britain, Japan and Eastern Europe, and bringing together a mass of evidence from the social and medical sciences, *Unhealthy Societies* provides the explanation. Healthy, egalitarian societies are more socially cohesive. They have a stronger community life and suffer fewer of the corrosive effects of inequality. The public arena becomes a source of supportive social networks rather than of stress and potential conflict.

As well as weakening the social fabric and damaging health, inequality increases crime rates and violence. *Unhealthy Societies* shows that social cohesion is crucial to the quality of life. Increased inequality imposes a psychological burden which reduces the well-being of the whole society. The pattern of modern disease shows that the material standard of living in developed countries is no longer the main issue. The problem is now the psycho-social quality of life, which must be supported by greater material equality. Without it, important social needs will go unmet and health will suffer. But this does not mean choosing between greater equity and economic growth; by lubricating the economy and society, investment in 'social capital' increases efficiency.

Richard Wilkinson is Senior Research Fellow at The Trafford Centre for Medical Research, University of Sussex.

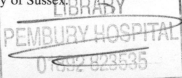

Unhealthy Societies

The Afflictions of Inequality

Richard Wilkinson

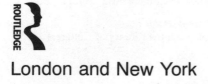

London and New York

9704166

WX 153

First published 1996
by Routledge
11 New Fetter Lane, London EC4P 4EE

Simultaneously published in the USA and Canada
by Routledge
29 West 35th Street, New York, NY 10001

Reprinted 1997, 1998

Typeset in Times by Keystroke, Jacaranda Lodge, Wolverhampton
Printed and bound in Great Britain by Clays Ltd, St Ives plc

British Library Cataloguing in Publication Data
A catalogue record for this book is available from the British Library

Library of Congress Cataloging in Publication Data
A catalog record for this book is available from the Library of Congress

ISBN 0–415–09234–5 (hbk)
ISBN 0–415–09235–3 (pbk)

Contents

Part V Redistribution, economic growth and the quality of life

Illustrations

TABLES

Preface

To have worked on the social and economic determinants of health for the last 20 years has been an enormous privilege. I first became involved when, after completing a Master's thesis, I wrote a newspaper article in the form of an open letter to the then Secretary of State for Health and Social Security, David Ennals, in Callaghan's Labour government in 1976.[1] Pointing out that, as a Labour minister, he presided over the largest social class differences in mortality then on record, I asked him to set up an 'urgent inquiry'. Three months later, after having read my article, he announced the setting up of the DHSS Working Group under the chairmanship of Sir Douglas Black. Three years later it produced the Black Report entitled *Inequalities in Health* and ushered in a new era of research on the social causes of health and illness throughout the developed world. Sir Douglas Black, who had been Chief Medical Officer in David Ennal's department, described his minister – with a characteristically neat turn of phrase – as 'a man who tried to do good and on the whole succeeded'.

The continuing research stimulated by this report is transforming our understanding of both society and health. Having started off with issues to do with the veracity of the basic figures, the progress of research has felt like a long and difficult climb, but we are now getting our first views of the landscape ahead. What we can see is destined to transform social and economic policy and hopefully, the direction of the social development of modern societies. It is now clear that the scale of income differences in a society is one of the most powerful determinants of health standards in different countries, and that it influences health through its impact on social cohesion. These basic facts have implications which go far beyond the health data from which they have emerged.

In many ways, doing research is like walking in the dark and trying to make out the dimly perceived shapes which loom up ahead of you. Initially, what you see is so unclear that you fear that it is as likely to be a product of your imagination, as of anything which actually exists. There is a natural desire to say what the shapes in the statistical darkness are as soon as possible. Balancing that is the fear that you will be proved wrong when the visibility increases. The result is sometimes nerve wracking. By great good fortune, the picture this book paints has been amply confirmed, while I have been writing it, by other researchers using independent data. Most recently, both Kaplan's group at Berkeley, and Kawachi's and Kennedy's at Harvard have shown that a society's life expectancy is closely related to the scale of income inequality within it. Even while writing this preface, I received a draft of another paper from the Harvard group in which they give a powerful statistical demonstration (correlations of 0.7 and 0.8) that income distribution is linked to social cohesion which, in turn, is linked to mortality.[2] Based on data from within the United States, this breakthrough removes any last doubts that I may have had about the discussion of socially cohesive societies and health in chapter 6.

This long journey – from social class differences in health to the effects of income distribution on social cohesion and national mortality rates – has not been without its traumatic episodes. But even when not embroiled in awful public rows, there have been long periods of sleepless worry over whether I may have made a fool of myself or led people up a blind alley. However, I have always felt part of a highly supportive – if geographically scattered – group of colleagues, who are able to express their concern, care and support for each other as we pursue our common endeavour. As well as enormously admiring the patience, thoughtfulness and thoroughness of their work, I would like to express my affection and gratitude to a wide group of friends working on the social and economic determinants of health on both sides of the Atlantic: in Sweden, The Netherlands, Germany, Canada and the United States, as well as in Britain. I owe most to people closer to home, particularly those associated with what have become known as the 'London' and 'Glasgow' groups, not to mention what may be a nascent Bristol group. I would love to go through all the names of those whose painstaking work is, I have no doubt, shaping a coming revolution in health and social policy. I owe my greatest debt to David Blane, Mel Bartley, Chris Power, Eric Brunner, Peter Townsend, Michael Marmot, Aubrey Sheiham, Yoav Ben-Shlomo and George Davey Smith. I hope I shall continue to learn from them and enjoy their friendship.

Closest to home is, of course, my family. Jenny Shaw has not only put up with my obsession with this subject – day and night – for so many years, but has endlessly given me the benefit of her expertise as a highly imaginative and creative academic sociologist, steering and developing my perceptions. She, like my extraordinarily loving children, George and Ann, has lived with my moods and carried me through periods when my work seemed to be collapsing around me and I felt like disappearing off the face of the earth.

More formally, I should like to acknowledge the financial support I have received from the Economic and Social Research Council, the Paul Hamlyn Foundation and the Lord Ashdown Charitable settlement. Lastly, I am constantly grateful to the staff of the library and the computing centre here at Sussex University, who have been unstinting with the practical help they have given me so many times over the years.

Brighton, April 1996

NOTES

1 Wilkinson, R.G. Dear David Ennals .... *New Society*, 16 December 1976; 567–8.
2 Kawachi, I., Kennedy B.P., Lochner, K., Prothrow-Stith, D. Social capital, income inequality, and mortality. *American Journal of Public Health* (forthcoming 1996).

Chapter 1

Introduction
The social economy of health

This book brings together a growing body of new evidence which shows that life expectancy in different countries is dramatically improved where income differences are smaller and societies are more socially cohesive. The social links between health and inequality draw attention to the fact that social, rather than material, factors are now the limiting component in the quality of life in developed societies.

The book starts out by asking why some societies are healthier than others. Having grown used to thinking about the determinants of individual health, researchers have given little attention to the broader question which policy-makers need answered. Yet the important factors which make some societies healthier than others may be quite different from those which differ between healthy and unhealthy individuals within the same society. It is, as so often, a matter of distinguishing the wood from the trees; but to do so means adopting a different vantage point.

The main impetus for taking a broader view of the determinants of health has come from research on health inequalities within developed countries. Research findings have increasingly focused attention on the wider features of the social and economic structure. As this field has developed, we have in effect been learning about the interface between the individual and society and the effects of structural factors on health: about how people are affected by social position, by wealth and poverty, by job insecurity and unemployment, by education, by social mobility; about why taller people move up the social hierarchy; about the importance of social networks; about family disruption; about stress at work and the social organisation of work. In doing so we have learned almost as much about society – or at least about how society impinges on the individual – as we have about health.

This book is an invitation to come on a rapid tour of the emerging picture of the interface between health and society. Over the last decade or two, pieces of the jigsaw have fallen into place increasingly rapidly – rather as they do when you are approaching the end of a puzzle and there are fewer pieces left to fill fewer spaces. It was not so long ago that people did not regard things like income and unemployment as belonging to an appropriate category to be called causes of health or illness. Medical advances of the past had seemed to have involved identifying single risk factors for single diseases: the broader concepts always seemed to have crumbled under closer scientific scrutiny. To people whose medical training had taught them to think about the effects of exposure to particular chemicals or germs, talk of social and economic structures affecting health sometimes seemed as remote as astrology. Even cigarettes were too broad a category: the 'real' cause of lung cancer was a particular fraction of tar or nicotine. But as people with backgrounds in the social sciences have moved into epidemiology (which studies health among populations instead of clinically in individuals), and medically trained epidemiologists have become more aware of the social sciences, increasing progress has been made on the wider picture.

Neither medical care nor genetics explains why one country is healthier than another, or why most countries gain two or three years of life expectancy with each decade that passes. Nor does it seem as if the big health differences between societies can be explained by adding up individual behavioural risk factors such as smoking, exercise and diet. Research has shown us that what matters is the nature of social and economic life. But what are the features which matter most? Some are easy to see: when we compare rich and poor countries no one doubts the importance of living standards. But why is life expectancy higher in countries like Greece, Japan, Iceland and Italy than it is in richer countries like the United States or Germany?

There is an important paradox at the heart of the relationship between health and living standards. Among the richer countries it looks as if economic growth and further improvements in living standards have little effect on health. They have advanced beyond a crucial stage in economic development when living standards reached a threshold level adequate to ensure basic material standards for all. This point is marked by the epidemiological transition when infectious diseases give way to the cancers and degenerative diseases as the main causes of death. During the same period, the so-called 'diseases of affluence' became the diseases of the poor in affluent societies.

The importance of the attainment of the threshold level of living standards marked by the epidemiological transition goes well beyond its significance for health. It marks a fundamental change in our relationship with economic growth and the nature of the benefits it has to offer us.

The other side of the paradox is that differences in the standard of living remain closely related to health *within* societies. That is to say, poorer people in developed countries may have annual death rates anywhere between twice and four times as high as richer people in the same society. It was the study of these dire health inequalities which made people aware of how important social and economic influences on health continued to be. Apparently regardless of the fact that health differences within societies remain so closely related to socioeconomic status, once a country had passed the threshold level of income associated with the epidemiological transition, its whole population can be more than twice as rich as another without being any healthier.

What is going on? And, if health inequalities were due to poverty, why have they got bigger in countries such as Britain during the last fifty years, despite huge rises in the standard of living?

If health is related to differences in living standards within developed societies, but not to the differences between them, we surely have to conclude that these differences mean something quite different within and between societies. Indeed, the evidence suggests that what matters within societies is not so much the direct health effects of absolute material living standards so much as the effects of social relativities. Health is powerfully affected by social position and by the scale of social and economic differences among the population. In terms of income, the relationship is with relative rather than absolute income levels.

The crucial evidence on this comes from the discovery of a strong international relationship between income distribution and national mortality rates. In the developed world, it is not the richest countries which have the best health, but the most egalitarian. Having been demonstrated by a number of different people using different data sets and different control variables, this relationship is now firmly established. But what is it about more egalitarian countries which makes them markedly healthier than less egalitarian ones? It is not simply that the poor use any additional income in more health-producing ways than the rich – say on better food rather than second cars. Not only does the relationship with income distribution hold even when controlled for the absolute incomes of the poor in a society, but if the poor used additional income more on necessities than on the luxuries bought by the rich, economic development might normally be expected to reduce health inequalities.

This relationship is important for several reasons. First, it appears to be one of the most powerful influences on the health of whole populations in the developed world to have come to light. Second, it seems to be closely related to health inequalities within countries. But beyond that, it has led to an understanding of the significance of the social fabric in developed societies.

Looking at a number of different examples of healthy egalitarian societies, an important characteristic they all seem to share is their social cohesion. They have a strong community life. Instead of social life stopping outside the front door, public space remains a social space. The individualism and the values of the market are restrained by a social morality. People are more likely to be involved in social and voluntary activities outside the home. These societies have more of what has been called 'social capital' which lubricates the workings of the whole society and economy. There are fewer signs of anti-social aggressiveness, and society appears more caring. In short, the social fabric is in better condition. The research tells us something very important about the way the social fabric is affected by the amount of inequality in a society.

Several features of the relationship between income distribution and national mortality rates fit this picture. Although all of the broad categories of causes of death – cardiovascular diseases, infections, respiratory diseases, cancers, etc. – seem to be related to income distribution, the most strongly related are social causes such as alcohol-related deaths, homicide and accidents. These causes are highly suggestive of the effects of social disintegration. The picture is reinforced by evidence of trends in crime and of growing social problems related to relative deprivation which affect children and young people in particular.

When looking at the nature of the pathways which are most likely to link physical disease to inequality, there are good reasons for thinking that psychosocial pathways are most important. Simply the fact that we are dealing with the effect of relative differences, rather than of absolute material standards, points strongly in that direction. The epidemiological evidence which most clearly suggests the health benefits of social cohesion comes from studies of the beneficial effects of social networks on health. People with more social contacts and more involvement in local activities seem to have better health, even after controlling for a number of other possibly confounding factors. But this is likely to be only part of the picture. Fortunately there is a large body of evidence demonstrating that various forms of psychosocial stress can have a powerful influence on death rates and rates of illness. The evidence comes from a wide variety of sources including randomised control trials, natural experiments and a range of other epidemiological observations. In addition there is increasing evidence of the physiological channels through which chronic stress can effect endocrine and immunological processes. There is even evidence showing that stressful social hierarchies predispose to poorer health among troops of baboons as well as in human societies. In addition some of the physiological pathways appear similar.

What comes out of this picture, pieced together as it is from the work of a large number of researchers, is enormously important. What it means is that the quality of the social life of a society is one of the most powerful determinants of health and that this, in turn, is very closely related to the degree of income equality. But that is only the beginning. The indications that the links are psychosocial make these relationships as important for the real subjective quality of life among modern populations as they are for their health. If the whole thing were a matter of eating too many chips or of not taking enough exercise, then that in itself would not necessarily mean that the quality of life which people experienced was so much less good. You can be happy eating chips. But sources of social stress, poor social networks, low self-esteem, high rates of depression, anxiety, insecurity, the loss of a sense of control, all have such a fundamental impact on our experience of life that it is reasonable to wonder whether the effects on the quality of life are not more important than the effects on the length of life. (We should note at this point that higher or lower life expectancy in this context is not primarily a matter of old people living a few years longer. More influential is the number of deaths at younger ages.) That the link between equity and health is largely a psychosocial link means that the scale of income differences and the condition of a society's social fabric are crucially important determinants of the real subjective quality of life among modern populations.

Health is telling us a story about the major influences on the quality of life in modern societies, and it is a story which we cannot afford to ignore. It addresses – in particular – the increasing disquiet about the contrast between the material success and social failure of modern societies. The extent to which the quality of life has been equated with the material standard of living is remarkable. This is no doubt partly because of the difficulty of measuring the social quality of life. Now, however, we know more about how crucial the nature of social life is and something of the dimensions that are important. On top of that, we also know that reducing income differences can improve matters.

This does not mean that we need abandon economic growth in favour of income redistribution. Indeed, the empirical evidence is that the narrower income differences associated with higher levels of social capital are likely to be beneficial to productivity. Rather than having to choose between equity and growth, it looks as if they have become complementary.

But it is not just that narrower income differences need not involve a sacrifice of growth. The puzzling relationship between life expectancy and Gross National Product per capita (GNPpc), as it changes over time, can be interpreted to mean that qualitative change is more important than quantitative growth, and that its benefits may hinge primarily on the cultural and social development which material progress loosely enables. Historically, growth has clearly been emancipating, enriching, and has added to human dignity. There are perhaps reasons to think that its emotionally civilising and socially liberating effects are not yet played out. If so, economic growth may still bring the indirect improvements in the social quality of life despite what has been said about threshold standards of living and the epidemiological transition.

Following this introduction, chapter 2 introduces the societal approach to health. It contrasts the approach to research and policy which comes from thinking about the determinants of individual health with the approach appropriate to a focus on overall health standards in population groups and societies. The distinction is not a matter of whether or not studies deal with large numbers of people. Indeed, most large health data sets are used to understand how health differs between individuals: they do not necessarily provide the most effective guide to the causes of the health differences between populations or the policies which would improve overall standards.

Chapter 3 discusses the reasons why life expectancy continues to rise in most developed countries by two or three years with every decade that passes. Although it seems as if this process must be closely associated with economic growth, the statistical relationship is very weak. The characteristics of the mismatch point to particular errors in the measurement of long-term changes in living standards and exclude a number of what might once have seemed plausible explanations of the health improvements. At the centre of this chapter is the explanation of the economic significance of the epidemiological transition. It is argued that the transition from infectious to degenerative causes of death marks the attainment of the minimum material standard consistent with health among the vast majority of the population. Thereafter, it looks as if absolute material standards cease to be the main obstacles to better health. This is consistent with the weak relationship between economic growth and increasing life expectancy, but it begs the question of the explanation for the continued rises in life expectancy.

Chapter 4 focuses on the important differences in health which remain associated with differences in living standards within each country. The chapter explains the data used to assess these differences and then goes on to show why they cannot be attributed to genetics; why only a small part is played by healthier people moving up the social ladder and the less healthy moving down; why almost none of the health differences results from differences in medical care; why the differences are only partly explained by health-related behaviour; and lastly, why the main explanations of health inequalities have to be found in the effects of the different social and economic circumstances in which people live.

Chapter 5 starts off from the apparent paradox that health is related to differences in living standards within developed societies but not to the differences between them. This inconsistency is resolved by evidence suggesting that what matters within countries is relative rather than absolute income levels. The chapter briefly summarises the evidence from different sources, showing that countries with narrower income differences tend to have lower average mortality rates. The possibility that it is a spurious relationship is discussed and dismissed. We then discuss, with the help of further research findings, how this relationship might be related to health inequalities within countries.

To help us interpret the relationship between income distribution and health, chapter 6 then looks for the common characteristics in five examples of societies which have been notably egalitarian and have had low mortality rates. The chapter starts off with Britain during the First and Second World Wars when civilian life expectancy increased unusually rapidly. It goes on to discuss Roseto, in Pennsylvania, which as well as being healthier than neighbouring towns was unusually closely knit. The chapter also considers an analysis of regional differences in Italy, the high standards of health which used to mark 'communist' countries, and the relative or absolute decline in health standards in Eastern Europe since about 1970. Finally it takes a brief look at Japan which simultaneously achieved an unusually narrow income distribution and the highest life expectancy in the world. In Roseto and Eastern Europe it is possible to see the loss of the health advantage associated with equity, while in Japan and wartime Britain it is possible to see that advantage being gained. The message that comes through clearly in each case is that the healthy, egalitarian countries have – or had – a sense of social cohesion and public spiritedness. Social rather than market values remained dominant in the public sphere of life.

Chapter 7 pursues the notion of social cohesion using material borrowed from anthropology and social psychology. It deals principally with how earlier forms of society used to order their economic life to ensure social harmony and minimise conflict. There is also some discussion of how market relations have a deep psychological effect on our experience of ourselves and our understanding of human relations.

Chapter 8 looks at the particular causes of death which are most symptomatic of particularly inegalitarian countries. As well as identifying a set of obviously 'social' causes indicative of social stress, it also notes statistical findings suggesting that higher crime rates, homicide and violence are associated with wider income differences. In addition, the chapter looks at several signs of increasing social malaise which accompanied the rapid widening of income differences in Britain during the later 1980s. In effect, this chapter is about the effects of social disintegration consequent on wider income differences, and stands in contrast to chapter 6.

Chapters 9 and 10 discuss the pathways through which inequality and loss of social cohesion are likely to affect health. The most important links are through the impact of psychosocial circumstances on health. Chapter 9 draws on numerous examples, using very different methods, to demonstrate the powerful impact which psychosocial circumstances have on physical health and on death rates. Chapter 10 deals with similar processes but at a more physiological level, looking particularly at the biological effects of chronic stress. The chapter shows some of the similarities between the effects of social hierarchy among baboons and among civil servants working in London. The chapter ends by describing some important recent research results showing the effects of psychosocial factors on children's growth which have powerful implications for their later emotional well-being and career chances.

Finally, chapter 11 puts all this together to paint a picture of the health and quality of life in modern societies as being primarily dependent on distributional justice and levels of what might be called 'social capital'. The extent of material inequality is a major determinant of psychosocial welfare in modern societies and its impact on health is but one of the social costs it carries with it. In essence the relationship between health and equity highlights the importance of human social needs and indicates the framework in which they can be satisfied. The chapter also draws attention to studies that suggest that, rather than being detrimental to growth, the gains in human functioning in more egalitarian societies lead to faster increases in productivity and higher growth rates. Chapter 11 also draws attention to the evidence that governments increase equity not when they are especially rich, as if it were a luxury which cannot normally be afforded, but instead when they face crises of legitimacy, or when they particularly need the population's co-operation, and can no longer afford to do without it.

Rather than implying that economic growth no longer brings real benefits to the developed world, it is suggested that its benefits are indirect rather than direct. The question is whether the mix of things that go into producing higher living standards increases or diminishes the social quality of life. We need to think of the indirect relationship between economic growth and the quality of life in much the same way as we might think about the indirect connection between material life and civilisation.

Part I

The health of societies

Chapter 2

Health becomes a social science

The remarkable two, three or even fourfold differences in death rates between different social classes or income groups which have come to light within most developed societies have served to remind people of the continued power of social and economic determinants of health. There has of course never been any doubt that the standard of living and extent of poverty were important determinants of health both in the Third World and at earlier stages of development in the developed countries. However, it was widely assumed that the growing affluence of the richer countries in the second half of the twentieth century meant that these influences on health had weakened their grip. It seemed understandable that social position would influence health when a substantial part of the population had difficulty in satisfying basic material needs; however, for social position to go on being so important when living standards were so much higher seemed to many to be highly implausible. In chapter 4 we will see why these differences cannot simply be 'explained away' and have to be taken at face value. Although the differences seemed to some to stretch credibility, the initial exploratory research has now been done and the conclusion is that the greater part of these health differences do indeed arise out of the social and economic fabric of life despite their failure to diminish under the impact of economic growth.

Our knowledge that people's social and economically structured life processes remain the most powerful influences on health in the modern world turns the exploration of the determinants of health into a social science. Medical science can address the biological pathways involved in disease, the pathology and the opportunities for treatment, but in so far as health is a social product and some forms of social organisation are healthier than others, advances in our understanding of health will depend on social research. The development of effective forms of prevention means understanding how social and economic structures impinge on people and what kinds of policies might be beneficial. It means understanding the implications of different institutional structures at work; of different forms of insecurity in relation to housing, income and jobs; of social and community development; it means understanding the determinants of the subjective quality of life; finding ways of strengthening the social fabric of society; above all, it means understanding the psychosocial effects of hierarchy and social position.

Two pieces of evidence stand out as indicators of the overwhelmingly social and political nature of population health. First is the range of diseases and causes of death which are more common lower down than further up the social scale. The lower-class health disadvantage is not explicable in terms of just one or two diseases which might be explained in terms of one or two risk factors. Death rates from about 80 per cent (83 per cent for men and 76 per cent for women) of the most important 80 or so causes of death (78 for men and 82 for women) are more common in blue-collar than white-collar workers. Every major group - infections, cancers, cardiovascular, nutritional and metabolic diseases, respiratory diseases, accidents, nervous and mental illnesses – shows the same pattern. Almost the only important diseases to show the opposite social gradient are skin cancer (resulting from overexposure to sun) and breast cancer. The very wide range of diseases that are related to social and economic status shows that we are dealing with a fundamentally social phenomenon: this is not merely the effect of the chance coincidence of a few health factors which tip the class gradient of disease one way rather than another.

Another quite different but almost equally striking indication of the importance of sociological processes are the health trends in Eastern Europe. If the countries of Eastern and Western Europe were arranged according to the rank order of their death rates in 1970, there would be a large area of overlap between countries of the two bloc. Eastern Germany did better than West Germany, while countries like Bulgaria and Romania did better than many Western European countries. If, however, they were lined up according to the death rates of men in 1990, all the countries in Eastern Europe did less well than all countries of Western Europe (Watson 1995), and death rates in Yugoslavia – which was in neither one camp nor the other – came exactly between the two political blocs. The national differences in women's mortality are only a little less clearly ordered. The change between 1970 and 1990 is not primarily a matter of the deteriorating mortality experience during the restructuring which followed the 1989 uprisings. From the early 1970s life expectancy throughout Eastern Europe ceased to improve. Having largely caught up with standards of life expectancy in Western Europe in the 1950s and 1960s, improvement ceased and a growing health gap opened up between Eastern and Western Europe – despite continued economic growth in most of Eastern Europe. The socio-political nature of the problem is suggested by the evidence that this failure cannot be explained in terms of straightforward issues like the declining standards of medical care, differential economic growth or increasing air pollution (Hertzman 1995). Something went wrong in all these societies at very much the same time in the early 1970s. Looking at the trends, it is hard to avoid thinking that if we understood what had prevented further progress in health, we would also have discovered the social and economic sources of the revolutions of 1989. As health and society are so closely related, learning about society tells us about health, and learning about health tells us about society.

An accurate overall conception of health has much in common with Durkheim's approach to suicide. Rather than analysing suicide purely in terms of individual psychology and circumstances, Durkheim saw suicide rates as a social product. Each society had a rate which reflected its social structure. When Durkheim was writing, much the most common cause of death was infectious disease, and it was clear that the incidence of infection had to be related primarily to exposure to infection and to material poverty. But if Durkheim had been writing now, it seems likely that in the context of the modern burden of disease in developed societies, he would not have confined his analysis to suicide. The evidence is overwhelming that the rates of most diseases vary from society to society in ways that reflect, and indeed are indicative of, differences in their social and economic organisation. Most of the main causes of death look no less sociological than suicide. No doubt Durkheim would have been particularly interested in the fact that the lack of progress in life expectancy in Eastern Europe from the early 1970s was much more marked among single than among married men and women. Mortality worsened substantially among single men and women during the 1970s and 1980s but changed little among the married (Watson 1995). This gives a powerful indication of how sociological are the underlying processes.

Looking at health from the standpoint of society rather than of individuals can lead to a radically different view of the determinants of health. Instead of looking to see what makes one individual healthier than another, our aim in this book will be to see what makes one *society* healthier than another. From the point of view of one's own personal health or the health of friends, understanding health differences between individuals will no doubt seem more relevant than understanding the health differences between societies. But from the point of view of practical politics and public policy, or indeed of its sociological interest, it is the health of whole societies which matters. The overriding issue is how to increase the sum total of health enjoyed by a society. From that perspective most of the health gains and losses going on among individuals in a society, whether to do with ageing, seasonal epidemics of infectious diseases, or the coming and going of other forms of illness, are little more than noise in the system. Very few individual health changes represent part of the processes that add to the total health of a society.

But surely the determinants of health identified in studies of individuals add up to become the societal determinants of health? Although the answer is in principal 'yes', in practice and from the point of view of research results, it may very well be that they do not. When what appears to be a determinant of health at the societal or group level of analysis is not confirmed as a risk factor in studies at the individual level of analysis, the societal finding tends to be labelled an 'ecological fallacy'. But there are reasons why individual and societal analyses may throw up different, but equally valid, results (Schwartz 1994; Susser 1994). A kernel of truth which shows up at the broader ecological level may easily escape statistical detection at the individual level. What really moves the health of whole societies, adding to or subtracting from the sum total of health, may be factors which account for only a very small part of the individual variation in health and so escape detection. Alternatively, factors responsible for major differences in the health of whole populations may be invariant among individuals within each society and so, once again, go undetected in studies of individuals. (Factors which affect everyone in a society uniformly are called constants and are invisible in statistical studies of individuals within that population because statistics is wholly concerned with analysing differences, or patterns of variation, among a large number of cases. The influence of a societal factor shared by everyone in a society could only be detected by making comparisons with different societies.) How often, one wonders, have potentially valuable findings been dismissed as ecological fallacies?

In practice, it looks as if some of the factors which seem to be important explanations of health differences between individuals do not account for the differences between social groups within societies or between one society and another. For instance, numbered among the healthiest countries in the world are countries with particularly high rates of smoking. This does not of course mean that smoking does not damage health: it means only that its influence is outweighed by other, usually unknown, factors which differ between one country and another. Similarly, fat consumption and cholesterol levels in Britain do not show the steep, social-class gradient that is found in heart disease. They affect individual risks of heart disease, but they are not among the things that differ systematically between social classes in ways that would contribute to the class gradient in disease.

There are also more fundamental problems in inferring from individual determinants of health to societal determinants. Both education and income appear to be important determinants of individual health. But one of the effects of having a good education is that it moves you up the social hierarchy. The improvement in health may be related to the change in individual social position which education effects rather than to education itself. If everyone in society suddenly had 25 per cent more education, it seems likely that it would improve health, but it might not. If social position is what matters and everyone's relative position remains unchanged, it would not. The same could be said of rises in income. Is it absolute or relative income that matters? Perhaps income only makes a difference if it improves your relative position in society. We shall see in chapter 5 that the evidence suggests that relative income matters more than absolute income. The same could be said of some of the research which shows that people with more social support have better health. If this was a reflection of a tendency for people with a more sociable personality to have better health regardless of their social environment, then better social relations in society as a whole might not improve overall health. Lastly, children taken to school by car may be protected from some of the dangers of the street, but each additional car journey increases air pollution and the danger of roads to others. Thus inferring to whole societies from studies of individuals could involve a kind of ecological fallacy in reverse. And from the point of view of changes in public policy, what matters is whether the results are right for society as a whole.

The extent to which societal issues do matter can be illustrated not merely by the obvious contrast between the health of developed and developing countries. In the years between 1965 and 1986 Japanese life expectancy increased by 7.5 years for men and 8 years for women. At the beginning of the period Japanese life expectancy was lower than in Britain. By the end of the period Japan had the highest life expectancy in the world. The order of magnitude of these gains can be seen from the fact that it would take the abolition of all heart disease and most cancers in Britain to achieve an equally large increase in British life expectancy (Marmot and Davey Smith 1989). However, it appears that these improvements cannot be explained in terms of changes in nutrition, health care, preventive health policies, or any of the obvious factors to have come out of individual studies.

Different levels of analysis produce different pictures of the determinants of health. As well as differences between individual and societal determinants, research on differences in the health of people grouped into social classes within the same society has focused attention on determinants of health which earlier had often been ignored. Studies suggest that the larger part of the social class differences in mortality cannot be explained by what seemed to be the important explanations for individual differences in health. Take, for example, the fourfold differences in death rates from heart disease found between senior and junior office workers working in government offices in Britain (see figure 4.1). Even after allowing for underestimation resulting from inaccurate measurements, all the major known individual risk factors for heart disease explain less than half of the difference (Marmot *et al.* 1978b). Several other studies have confirmed that social class gradients in 'all cause' mortality remain almost as steep after controlling for the effects of major individual risk factors.

Adding weight to the reasons for tackling the determinants of health at a societal level is the sociological patterning of risk exposure to which Rose drew attention (Rose 1992). His argument in favour of a societal approach was not concerned with possible differences between the factors that are important at the individual and societal levels. Instead, he argued that many of the factors recognised as important at the individual level required intervention at the societal level. Essentially, because behaviour is socially determined, individuals can only be changed by changing society. Rather than regarding people with a particular disease or exposed to some risk factor as individuals who differ in some categorical way from the rest of the normal population, Rose showed their numbers were given by the characteristics of the whole population. Rather than the sick being divided from the rest of the population by a clear discontinuity, they represent one end of a continuous population distribution. One of the first examples of this pattern which came to light was high blood pressure. People with hypertension turned out not to be a distinct group added on to the top end of the normal distribution of blood pressure in society. Instead of having some specific defect absent in the rest of the population, they come within the range of variability described by the bell-shaped curve of the normal distribution. The same appears to be true for a number of other risk factors for heart disease, including high cholesterol levels.

After looking at the distribution of risk factors in thirty-two different countries at all levels of economic development, Rose concluded that the proportion of people at high risk in any population is simply a function of the *average* blood pressure, cholesterol levels or whatever in that society. His evidence suggested that this was true for a number of conditions. Thus the proportion of the elderly population who suffer senile dementia seems to be a function of the level of cognitive ability of the whole population. Likewise the number of heavy drinkers is closely predicted by the average alcohol consumption per head of population; while the prevalence of obesity is closely related to the average ratio of weight to height. Indeed, Rose claims that this is also true of measures of depression, mental health and aggression.

Although the overall variation in any population will include the effects of genetic variation, the way in which the whole population distribution of these conditions is shifted up or down in different societies reflects differences in the society's way of life. Rose interpreted his evidence as showing that you could not reduce the proportion of the population at high risk on a wide range of risk factors without reducing the whole society's exposure to that risk. In effect, the extent of the variation round a society's norms is fixed so that the proportion of people with bad diets, who are heavy drinkers, have high blood pressure, etc. is a reflection of where the society's norms are. Rose's evidence suggested that it was easier to change the societal norms than to leave them unchanged while trying to reduce the proportion of the population over some level of risk.

None of this may seem very surprising given that many characteristics and features of human behaviour will be normally distributed within each society – partly reflecting patterns of social cohesion. But it does conflict with the common idea of disease as an autonomous individual affliction. It emphasises the extent to which modern diseases and the underlying exposures to a wide range of risk factors are a product of the norms of the society in which we live. The apparent strength of the sociological determination of individual disease led Rose to conclude that preventive policy had to be directed, not towards people in the unhealthy tail of the population distribution, but towards moving the entire distribution of behaviour/practice/exposure among the population as a whole. To reduce deaths from cirrhosis, for example, we would all have to drink less. As heavy drinkers differentiate themselves from the norm, the frequency of drinking which constitutes the norm will determine how many people become alcoholics. This amounts to saying that processes of differentiation are more fundamental than the norms around which differentiation takes place. Rose quotes Dostoevsky: 'We are all responsible for all.'

This relates to the conclusions which Syme drew from the very limited success which attempts to reduce individual behavioural risk factors have had. He described the problem in the context of the disappointing results of the Multiple Risk Factor Intervention Trial (MRFIT) in the United States (Syme 1996). Men in the highest 10 per cent of risk for coronary heart disease – who might therefore be regarded as highly motivated – were only persuaded to make minimal changes in their eating and smoking despite six years of intensive attempts to persuade them to change. Syme commented:

> even when people do successfully change their high risk behaviors, new people continue to enter the at-risk population to take their place. For example, every time we finally helped a man in the MRFIT project to stop smoking, it is probable that, on that day, one or two children in a school yard somewhere were for

the first time taking their first tentative puffs on a cigarette. So, even when we do help high risk people to lower their risk, we do nothing to change the distribution of disease in the population because . . . we have done nothing to influence those forces in the society that caused the problem in the first place.

(Syme 1996, p. 22)

This is an additional reason for taking a societal approach to health. But it has implications for policy, as well as for the research needed to guide it, which go well beyond the problems of tackling coronary risk factors. Studies of individuals and social groups typically come up with sharply contrasting policy implications. Studies of individuals lead constantly to attempts to distinguish between people with and without some problem (some disease or social problem) who all belong to the same population or social group. The approach is to identify people with symptoms of the disease and then find out what is – or was – different about their lifestyle or socioeconomic circumstances. Almost invariably, the result is that you identify a group of people 'at high risk' of the disease, identified because they have particular vulnerability factors or whatever, and the problem then becomes one of how to intervene amongst this group to prevent them getting the disease. Sometimes it is a matter of providing screening and early treatment, other times of trying to change some aspect of lifestyle, but always it is a matter of providing some service or intervention. This applies not just to health, but also to studies of a wide range of social, psychological, developmental and educational problems. What happens is that the original source of the problem in society is left unchanged (and probably unknown) while expensive new services are proposed to cater for the individuals most affected. Each new problem leads to a demand for additional resources for services to try to put right the damage which continues to be done. Because the underlying flaw in the system is not put right, it gives rise to a continuous flow, both of people who have suffered as a result, and of demands for special services to meet their needs.

But another approach is possible. Take, for example, the high adolescent suicide rates in Japan. They might have been tackled by identifying those at risk and then providing expensive counselling services in every school and college; but over the years suicides have declined very dramatically in the 15–20 and 20–25 year age groups, especially among boys, without such services. Instead, changes in the educational system have made students' paths through it more predictable and reduced the likelihood of unrealistic illusions and resulting disappointments (Dore 1995). The changes were both cheaper and more effective than additional services would have been. In the occupational sphere, job stress provides another example. Instead of providing expensive counselling services for employees in high-stress situations, companies might find that changes in office practice could reduce sickness absence and increase productivity (Karasek and Theorell 1990). Instead of responding to job stress in ways that increased costs, a more radical approach might not only have avoided the cost of additional services, but perhaps even have increased efficiency.

There are then a number of different reasons for thinking that much more attention needs to be given to the societal determinants of health. They fall under two headings. In terms of research, the explanations of what makes whole populations healthier than others may be very different from the evidence which comes out of studies of what makes some individuals healthier than others. In addition, there is clear evidence that there are societal determinants of health to be identified. Then in terms of policy: first, even when it comes to tackling the individual risk factors, it may sometimes be more effective to tackle them at a societal level; and second, if prevention is not to depend on a continuous stream of expensive new services to cope with people identified as high risk, it will have to tackle the environment that establishes levels of exposure to risk.

In almost every sphere of social policy we imagine that services and interventions are more important than they are. Not only is the influence of medical services on survival dwarfed (as we shall see in the next chapter) by the influence of social and economic circumstances, but police and prisons have only a minor impact on crime; social workers cannot solve society's social problems; remedial teachers cannot – in two hours per week – offset the effects of emotional trauma in a child's background; community development workers cannot make communities, and family therapists cannot prevent families falling apart. Evaluations in all these areas provide evidence of what is, at best, only marginal effectiveness.

If the health risks to which people are differentially exposed arose merely from the material circumstances in which we live, that would tell us very little about our society which we could not see with our own eyes. What makes understanding health sociologically important is that many modern health problems reflect people's subjective experience of the circumstances in which they live. This is because many of the crucial pathways leading to disease are, as we shall see, psychosocial. The psychological repercussions of social circumstances are known to contribute to morbidity and mortality from a wide range of conditions. The implication is that the disease profile of different societies, and of different status groups within populations, tells us something about the subjective impact of social and economic systems. It means that health can provide new clues to the subjective tenor of society.

The analysis of the socioeconomic determinants of death rates is a particularly important guide to understanding social welfare, not merely because the criteria are clear and the records complete. It is also important because the social determinants of health provide essential insights into the way social structures impose psychic damage and human costs. Health, as we shall see, gives us a handle of hard data on the subjective impact of experience. In many areas of social welfare, measurement is beset with problems of shifting definitions and criteria, of not knowing whether changes in the numbers represent real changes or merely changes in reporting or recording. Lastly, the sociology of health has the advantage that people's understanding of what causes ill-health is less dominated by ideas of blame and punishment than it is in some other areas of social functioning.

The difficulty is to identify and implement the institutional changes that would tackle problems at root. There is of course a long history of legal safeguards and reforms dealing with hazards that could be avoided by a quick technological fix: such as limiting exposure to toxic materials or putting guards on machines. While there are always complaints about the costs, and last-ditch criticisms of the evidence from those whose financial interests are threatened, technical solutions have made major contributions to occupational and environmental health. But what is now coming out of health research, and particularly health inequalities research, is knowledge of the social causes of disease. Instead of exposures to toxic materials and mechanical dangers, we are discovering the toxicity of social circumstances and patterns of social organisation. We know very well that if the threefold differences in death rates which have been shown to exist between senior and junior office workers (Marmot *et al.* 1984) arose as a result of exposure to toxic materials, the affected offices would be closed down immediately until the problem was solved. Similarly, if the fourfold difference in death rates recorded between people living in richer and poorer neighbourhoods of the Northern Region of England (Phillimore *et al.* 1994) were traced to factory pollutants, people would be evacuated while an emergency clean-up operation was organised. However, fortunately for the vested interests which would be threatened, neither the social causes nor their devastating effects on mortality are well known. But, given how recently health inequalities went almost unrecognised and the rate at which knowledge of their causes is advancing, there are grounds for thinking that during the next decade or so these issues may provide the impetus for a new era of social reform.

In many areas of research statistics provide a kind of social microscope. They show features of social reality and relationships between things which are invisible to a naked eye. If you mentioned social class differences in death rates twenty years ago, even to doctors or others concerned with health care, the first question was often, 'Which way round are they?' The fact that lower-class death rates were at least twice as high as upper-class ones was socially invisible. Although we can all see that there are more elderly women than elderly men, and know that this is because of survival differences, we are not aware that there is an even greater imbalance between the number of upper- and lower-class elderly people arising from the survival differences over the life course. It has taken years of research which has statistically demonstrated these relationships, and continuous media items relaying their findings to a wider public, to make them 'visible'. Public understanding of the social determinants of health has grown rapidly over the last two decades. Everyone now knows that the poor have worse health and a shorter life expectancy than the rich.

Whereas the causes of the sex differences in survival are likely to be largely biological, the causes of the class differences are primarily a matter of the different socioeconomic circumstances in which people live. In the past governments have tended to use the lack of knowledge of the precise causes as an excuse for their inaction, but it is an excuse which grows progressively thinner. If the relationship between health and deprivation was as clearly understood as the relationship between fuel poverty and deaths among the elderly from hypothermia, the demand for action would be difficult to resist. In Britain, news media across the political spectrum have demanded action on hypothermia with the result that a most recalcitrant government had first to institute a system of additional cold-weather payments for pensioners to pay for extra heating, and then to compensate pensioners and others on low incomes for the addition of value added tax to fuel prices. As research on the socioeconomic determinants of health progresses, and public understanding of the issues increases, the demand for social reform will become unstoppable. Growing knowledge changes both the morality and the rationality of the status quo. It turns excusable official inaction into culpable negligence.

This area has the potential to provide the basis of a reform of the social environment equivalent to the reforms of the physical environment brought about by the public health movement initiated in the Victorian era. Just as the benefits of those reforms extended beyond health into the quality of life, so the social reforms necessitated by a recognition of the social determinants of health will improve the quality of life as well as health.

The usual proxy for a measure of the quality of life is of course income. But instead of providing the empirical evidence, as health does, of how human beings are affected by the quality of the social, economic and material environment, the meaning of income comes from our tendency to believe, as part of the economic catechism of our society, that it is the means to human self-realisation: that self-fulfilment can be bought. At a societal level, because income gives everyone greater freedom and power to pursue whatever they want, a society's richness is used as the next best thing to a measure of its goodness. In the absence of good measures of other aspects of human welfare, the fact that income provides an accurate measure of our power to consume means that, encouraged by economists, we slip into a tendency to think that rather than being a necessary precondition of life, consumption is what life is about. Too often economic theory seems to suggest either that we have an innate desire to maximise consumption or that it is the only aim granted the accolade of 'rational' behaviour. At the population level, however, income and health provide rather different definitions of the 'good society'. The most important difference between them seems to be that income ignores the importance of social life which health emphasises.

Several attempts have been made to improve on Gross National Product per capita (GNPpc) as a measure of a society's welfare. So-called 'Measures of Economic Welfare' have been produced which, amongst other things, take out of national income some of the economic ills, like air pollution or car crashes, which necessitate increased expenditure without adding to net welfare (Daley and Cobb 1990; Jackson and Marks 1994). But despite such efforts, income will always have two major failings as a basis on which to measure welfare. The first is that it is fundamentally incapable of measuring qualitative change. As products develop over the years and new kinds of products appear on the market, there is no way in which economic indices can adequately assess their changing significance for welfare. Monetary indices could provide an adequate summary of increased wealth only if the process of economic growth – by which we get richer – simply brought us more of exactly the same range of goods and services which our parents and grandparents enjoyed. Because most of the transformation wrought by economic development involves qualitative change, not only in consumption but in every aspect of the way we live, most of what is important escapes the attention of monetary indices. Even the basis of something as apparently simple as a Retail Price Index is stymied by the constant process of qualitative change in the goods and services we use (Siegal 1994).

The second failing of Measures of Economic Welfare is that, as their name implies, they leave out social welfare. The enormous social changes which come in on the back of economic development are all-important to human welfare. Even before societies have risen above basic minimum subsistence standards, people's welfare is crucially dependent on the social environment. In the developed nations, where basic material standards for the vast majority of the population are well above the minimum, social welfare becomes a larger part of the picture.

The ability of health research to illuminate important issues of social welfare and the quality of life does not rest on *a priori* assumptions. Health is sensitive to qualitative and quantitative changes in material and social life. If it turned out that good health was simply a matter of avoiding chocolate and chips and a few other attractive vices – sloth, gluttony, idleness, etc. – then it would seem that in some important respects health was related inversely to the quality of life. For many, health would appear to involve a sacrifice of happiness. However, research has shown that health is highly sensitive – not only to happiness itself – but also to specific aspects of social welfare. The psychosocial pathways through which health is affected means that it is able to provide a window on subjective psychosocial experience and show us how we are affected by important features of social organisation. We shall look at the evidence for this in chapters 6, 8 and 9.

Research is increasingly able to document the human costs of particular features of the social and economic structure of modern societies. In particular, the underlying causes and pathways responsible for the excess mortality which occurs in less privileged sections of society are becoming clearer. Not unexpectedly, their broad outlines have much in common with the likely sources of a number of other social problems – including emotional disturbance in childhood, poor educational performance, crime and violence.

The problems associated with deprivation impose additional costs on society in numerous different ways. They do this in part through the need for additional services – whether this is a matter of growing prison populations, additional medical services, of dealing with more classroom conflict in schools, the costs of drug addiction, social services or whatever. Costs are also imposed through the need for social security payments to people demoralised or incapacitated by their social circumstances and lack of educational and job opportunities. As well as public costs, there are also private costs such as the improved security systems – locks, alarms and constant vigilance – needed to protect property, or the human costs associated with fear of street violence and the restrictions on personal freedom which it creates.

All these costs, whether public or private, financial or social, are the costs of dealing with the symptoms, rather than the causes, of the social failure of modern societies. The reluctance to countenance changes in the socioeconomic structures which create these problems leads to a build-up of costs attributable to the lack of reform of the social structure. We pay for not making changes and presumably what we pay is the price of the growing contradictions which at some stage must bring about change in the prevailing social system. Essentially this is the source of the crisis in the welfare state which confronts so much of the developed world.

Unreformed, the social and economic structure creates problems which impose cost burdens on the whole society, particularly on the public sector. This burden, and the waste of the human resources of a large minority of the population which goes with it, severely impairs economic performance and competitiveness. Poorer economic performance not only deepens and widens the extent of a . society's social failure by pushing up unemployment and relative poverty, but it also reduces a nation's ability to meet the costs of that failure. As an increasing proportion of the population is relegated to relative poverty, people are turned from being net contributors to a society's welfare to being a net burden on it. This, in turn, further threatens prosperity, so confirming the vicious circle which both increases the social burden and curtails the society's ability to respond effectively to it. International evidence, which we shall review briefly in chapter 11, shows that rather than having to choose between equity and economic growth, in a modern economic system greater equity is now associated with faster growth.

If the only kind of reform which policy-makers can envisage is to add expensive services in a battle to keep abreast of growing social damage, then politicians will believe that there is no solution: political parties of neither the left nor the right are likely to believe they can afford major increases in public expenditure: demands for additional services will fall on deaf ears. Nor is the solution to cut benefits and services while maintaining the system which creates the need for them. From the societal point of view, such cuts will be offset by rising social costs. The real solution is to identify more fundamental changes which incur only the initial costs of making the necessary preventive changes in the institutional structures.

International comparisons show that there are very important differences in the scale of social problems which different countries face. On the one hand there are countries like the USA, and increasingly Britain, with high crime rates, large prison populations, low educational standards, high health inequalities and relatively poor overall standards of health. On the other hand there are countries like Japan and Sweden which – at least until the late 1980s – had low crime rates, low health inequalities, high educational standards and the highest life expectancy in the world. Such differences show that the basic social and economic system which all these countries have in common, has been made to work a great deal better in some countries than in others. Indeed, it testifies to the overall importance of getting the relationship between economy and society right.

Chapter 3

Rising life expectancy and the epidemiological transition

Neither of the two most striking features of population health is properly understood. There is no adequate explanation of the upward trend in life expectancy and standards of health which continues in most countries of the world, and we still do not understand why health varies so dramatically with differences in socioeconomic status within each country. In this chapter we shall discuss the first of these issues. The differences in health within societies comprise the subject of the next chapter.

Throughout most of the world, life expectancy continues to improve from one generation to the next. In the developed world two to three years are added to life expectancy at birth with each decade that passes. This is much the most important process affecting human health both nationally and internationally, yet we have very little knowledge of its causes. As we shall see, none of the assumed explanations, such as the development of medical science, public health measures and the benefits of economic growth, fits at all well. Indeed, it is only as we have come to see what is wrong with such explanations that we have become aware of what a fundamental gap there is in our knowledge. Although most developed countries have been enjoying the benefits of almost continuous increases in life expectancy for at least a century, we lack theories that even begin to fit the data.

It is perhaps worth noting at the outset, that while the increases in life expectancy are largely responsible for the dramatic increases in the proportion of old people in developed countries, this is not primarily because increasing life expectancy has made old people live longer. Although people in their seventies and eighties do live a little longer than they used to, the main improvements have come from a reduction of death rates at earlier ages. Broadly speaking, the younger the age group, the greater has been the reduction in death rates. The biggest decline has been in infant mortality, followed by large reductions in childhood mortality, and progressively smaller declines amongst younger and older adults. So although death rates of people in their seventies and eighties have changed least since last century, a much higher proportion of people now survives to old age.

We shall start out by looking at the causes of the historical rise in life expectancy and then go on to discuss what might lie behind current trends.

The bulk of the decline in death rates since last century in the developed countries has been a decline in mortality from infectious diseases. (That the more recent decline is principally a decline in mortality from non-infectious degenerative diseases is one important reason for keeping the past and present separate in this discussion.) In his highly influential work, McKeown pointed out that the vast bulk of the decline in mortality from infectious diseases came before medicine had effective forms of treatment or immunisation (McKeown *et al.* 1975). He argued that this meant that the change was not the result of the application of medical science. Death rates came tumbling down during the later nineteenth century onwards. Theoretically, Jenner's use of cowpox to vaccinate (the word comes from *vacca* meaning cow) against smallpox from as early as 1796 means that the decline in mortality from smallpox could have been an exception where medicine *did* make a difference. However, the downward trend in deaths looks much like that in other diseases for which vaccination was not available, and there seems no reason for thinking that vaccination made more than a minor contribution to a downward trend which was driven by the same underlying factors as the decline in mortality from other diseases.

The fact that medical science cannot explain most of the decline in mortality from the infections is not of course evidence that medical care is ineffective. It means that in this instance its effectiveness came too late to account for anything more than the tail end of the decline in infectious mortality. However, estimates of the current contribution of modern medical care to the growth of life expectancy in the developed world do not suggest that it can explain very much of the continuing increase in life expectancy. The most generous recent estimate based on an analysis of major medical procedures, including medical forms of prevention such as screening and immunisation, suggests that the whole modern medical effort adds no more than about five years' difference to modern life expectancy (Bunker *et al.* 1994). Most of this comes from treatment rather than prevention. There are other indicators which suggest that medicine may play a substantially smaller role than this. Even among those causes of death where medical treatment is most effective, the social and economic determinants of mortality remain substantially more powerful (Mackenbach *et al.* 1990).

The common assumption that the provision of clean water supplies and sewers accounts for past improvements in health ignores the fact that the bulk of the decline in mortality has been from airborne rather than waterborne diseases. However, we should note that Szreter (1988) has argued that public health measures may have been important beyond the confines of waterborne diseases partly because any measures which reduced the combined onslaught of disease on our immune systems would probably have made us better able to cope with other infections.

A few diseases such as cholera were almost entirely eliminated. Tuberculosis might have been added to that category if it were not for the recent upturn associated with the increase in poverty during the 1980s. What has happened among most of the other great infectious killers of the nineteenth century (such as whooping cough, flu, diphtheria, measles and scarlet fever) is that although, if not immunised, we can still continue to catch them, they have gradually become less severe diseases. Several have become normal childhood infections with an almost negligible mortality (in so far as any child mortality can ever be called 'negligible'). We all continue to get new varieties of flu, but they are only regarded as lifethreatening among the frail elderly. The problem is to understand why these diseases became less serious. Did human resistance increase or did the virulence of the infective organisms decline? Did we change or did they?

After excluding explanations in terms of medical care, McKeown plumped for increases in the standard of living, particularly improved nutrition and housing, as the most likely explanation of the weakening effect of the infectious diseases. He produced no direct statistical or other evidence of an association, but arrived at this conclusion as the only thing left after having excluded other explanations along the lines outlined above (McKeown *et al.* 1975). He discussed the possibility that the infectious organisms may have evolved less virulent forms but concluded that, although it is a possibility in one or two cases, it is unlikely to be the main explanation. As well as the argument he uses on that point, one needs to remember that many of these diseases went on being major killers in poorer countries – presumably not because they had quite different strains.

One possibility that McKeown does not consider seriously is that human beings became less susceptible for genetic rather than environmental reasons. Diseases with very high mortality in childhood and infancy will exert a very powerful selective effect, killing a large proportion of those most susceptible before they can grow up and pass their genes on to the next generation. Although the era during which we were exposed to high death rates was not long enough to have selected new genetic mutations conferring higher levels of resistance to these diseases, it may well have been long enough to establish a population bred selectively from the parts of the genetic variation existing in the population where resistance was highest. Because the highest mortality rates from these diseases were in childhood, the most vulnerable members of the population would not have lived to have children. If the population's initial gene pool had contained a proportion of people with immune systems capable of throwing off these infections, the genes of these people would have quickly increased their frequency in the population, generation by generation.

It might be possible to test such an explanation by modelling each disease mathematically in the population. The initial case-survival rate could be used as an indicator of how frequently an adequate level of resistance occurred among the population. How quickly this was preferentially selected to form the breeding stock of the next generation would be given by the mortality rate for that disease among the population below reproductive age. These calculations could be checked against a predicted decline in the case-fatality rate in the next generation. It would then be possible to see if the shape of the curve of declining mortality was consistent with such an explanation.

Some of this kind of infectious disease modelling has been done on diseases in other species (such as myxomatosis among rabbits), but it has not been done among human populations. However, Burnet gives some striking evidence from other societies of declining case-fatality rates in the absence of economic development – which has the advantage of excluding the rising standard of living as a rival explanation (Burnet and White 1972). There is a widespread tendency for diseases which have been recently introduced into populations to have very high mortality rates. European migrants to other continents in previous centuries brought diseases which more than literally decimated indigenous population. Similarly, the migrants themselves succumbed in large numbers to the diseases they first met in other countries. After a few generations case-fatality rates usually begin to fall. Burnet mentions the example of tuberculosis in Mauritius where, he says, it takes 'something over a hundred years after its first contact with tuberculosis for a race to develop a resistance against the disease equivalent to that of a European population' (ibid.: 219). He says the pattern was much the same for tuberculosis among American Indians.

However, the fact that we have seen signs of the re-emergence of tuberculosis with the recent growth of poverty in some of the developed countries suggests that there must be an important environmental component in the decline of infections. In addition, unless modern standards of life expectancy were sustained by modern living standards, there would be no reason why death rates should have sunk below those which were normal in previous centuries. A theory of genetic selection would be most suitable for explaining a slow return to 'normal' mortality levels after a sudden rise in mortality caused by the introduction of a new disease. What we see, however, is a decline of all infectious causes of mortality after infectious diseases had been the dominant causes of mortality for very many more centuries than the hundred years which Burnet suggests had been enough for genetic selection to lower TB death rates in Mauritius. So, because the historical pattern is not so much a matter of getting over a temporary upsurge in infectious mortality before returning to pre-existing death rates, but is instead a reduction of infectious mortality of all kinds to levels unknown in any earlier historical periods, the primary place must be given to the rising standard of living.

We shall now move on to see what might lie behind the continuing improvement in health standards in the modern world. The broad picture is shown in figure 3.1. It sets out the relationship between Gross National Product per capita (GNPpc) and life expectancy at birth for men and women combined among countries at all stages of development. Each point is a country, and the four curves show the relationship between GNPpc and life expectancy as it was in 1900, 1930, 1960 and 1990.

Life expectancy (years)

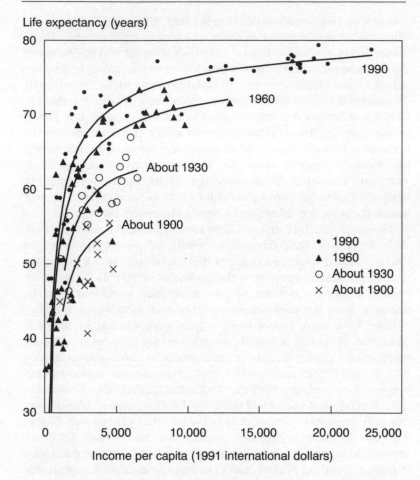

Figure 3.1 Life expectancy and income per capita for selected countries and periods
Source: World Bank, *World Development Report*, 1993

At lower levels of GNPpc there was, at each point in time, an apparent relationship with life expectancy in that the two seem to rise together. However, at higher levels of GNPpc the relationship seems to disappear: at each point in time the curve flattens out towards the horizontal. This suggests that once countries have reached some threshold level of income (around $5000 per capita in 1990), life expectancy plateaus out and further increases in GNPpc are no longer associated with increases in life expectancy.

However, an addition of (say) $500 per capita is only a very small percentage increase in the incomes of rich countries, though a very substantial one in poor countries. One might ask whether the same percentage increase in income in rich and poor countries would have a more uniform impact on life expectancy. This possibility can be examined very simply by taking the log of GNP per capita. On this basis it appears that life expectancy has something much nearer a linear relationship with proportionate increases in GNPpc. This means that the doubling of income from say $1,000 to $2,000 a year per capita buys the same number of additional years' life expectancy as the doubling of income from say $10,000 to $20,000. The fact that in absolute terms the same number of years' increase in life expectancy costs $1,000 per capita in poorer countries and $10,000 in richer ones shows a pattern at any given date of very sharply diminishing health returns to increases in income. In fact, at higher levels of development the improvements in life expectancy seem to fall significantly below the log linear trend showing even more sharply diminishing health returns to increases in income (Wilkinson 1994a).

If we could see only the 1990 curve in figure 3.1 it might be thought that life expectancy fails to rise further because it had reached close to some upper limit of longevity for human populations. But even without the perspective given to us by the earlier curves, there are a number of reasons for thinking that this is not the case. First is the recent tendency for developed countries with high life expectancies to show falls in death rates even at older ages. This trend has become more marked partly as a result of the largely unexplained decline in heart disease. Second, in those countries whose health inequalities have widened, death rates are falling fastest among those social strata which already have the highest life expectancy. If we were running into the buffer of some upper limit to life expectancy, one might expect it to lead to a universal narrowing of health inequalities as the poor caught up with the rich who had already arrived at the buffers. Needless to say, no such pattern is yet evident.

However, the most important reason for thinking that the levelling off of the curves in figure 3.1 has nothing to do with reaching some absolute biological limits of human life expectancy is the fact that, even among nations on the horizontal part of the curve, life expectancy continues to rise with the passage of time by an average of two or three years for every decade that passes. But perhaps we should instead regard it as an indication that there may be limits to human life expectancy within any given historical context.

Looking at the curves for different data in figure 3.1 it is clear that life expectancy increases not so much by countries moving out along a given curve, but by moving on to new, higher curves. Indeed, as early as 1975 Preston concluded that no more than 12 per cent of the improvement in life expectancy was associated with the rising standard of living (Preston 1975).

In order to get a clearer idea of whether health really is responsive to rising living standards among the rich countries on the flat part of figure 3.1, let us move from cross-sectional data to look at changes over time. Figure 3.2 shows the relationship between percentage changes in GNPpc and changes in life expectancy over the twenty years 1970-90 among the rich market countries belonging to the Organisation for Economic Cooperation and Development (OECD). Among these countries it is possible to compare GNPpc at purchasing power parities rather than according to the vagaries of changing exchange rates between currencies. This means that pounds, francs, yen, etc. are converted into dollars according to the comparative cost of the same basket of goods in each country. In other words, the changes in GNPpc shown in figure 3.2 are more accurate reflections of changes in real purchasing power in each country. The twenty-year span over which change is measured means that comparisons are less likely to be upset by unknown lag periods between changes in GNPpc and life expectancy.

As if to confirm Preston's findings, figure 3.2 also shows no more than a very weak relationship between life expectancy and GNPpc. The correlation between the changes is 0.3. This suggests again that no more than about 10 per cent of the variation in the rate of increase in life expectancy is related to variations in the rate of increase in GNPpc. This conclusion almost exactly echoes Preston's, despite the fact that his was based on an analysis of data some twenty years earlier. In effect it means that one country can achieve economic growth rates twice as high as another over a twenty-year period without necessarily showing more substantial improvements in life expectancy.

It appears then that as much as 90 per cent of the modern increases in life expectancy enjoyed in the rich countries is not closely enough associated with economic growth to produce correlations with long-term rates of growth. Analysis suggests that around 10 per cent of the improvements in life expectancy come

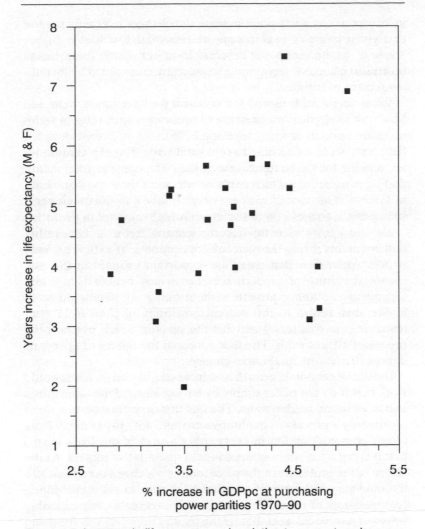

Figure 3.2 Increase in life expectancy in relation to percentage increase in GDPpc. OECD countries, 1970–90
Sources: OECD *National Accounts*, Paris, 1992 and World Bank, *World Tables*, 1992

from moving out along a curve of rising real incomes, while most of the remaining 90 per cent comes from moving from lower to higher curves shown in figure 3.1.

In this context it is interesting to note that while the flattening cross-sectional curves show diminishing health returns to increases in income at any given point in time, the changes over time suggest that given levels of real income are associated with ever higher levels of health-increasing returns. In effect, diminishing health returns to income at any point in time are accompanied by increasing returns over time.

What does all this mean? It looks as if we have largely removed McKeown's residual explanation of declining death rates in terms of rising incomes among developed countries in recent decades, but so far we have nothing to replace it with. The explanation we are looking for has to function as a kind of income gearing factor; that is, as something which explains why over time, the same level of GNPpc is associated with ever higher levels of life expectancy, so causing us to move on to successively higher curves in figure 3.1.

No one knows what this income gearing factor is. One rather dull possibility is that the measures of economic growth are simply wrong. Another is that there are important changes in the psychosocial culture of modern societies which benefit health and accompany economic growth without being intimately linked to it. We shall return to this second possibility in chapter 11 after discussing (in chapters 9 and 10) the ways in which psychosocial processes affect health. The first concerns the failure of economic indices to measure qualitative change.

Indices of economic growth and increases in real incomes would work best if we got richer simply by having more of the same things as our Victorian predecessors. The fact that economic development is primarily a process of qualitative change, not only in every facet of our consumption but in every other aspect of our lives, means that it is not adequately summarised in quantitative indices. At the centre of the problem are the price indices which are used to deflate the monetary measures of incomes or output to get 'real' values, real measures of output per head or real increases in purchasing power. They would work best if the quality of goods was fixed and you could simply see how the prices of each item – say coats, cars, domestic fuel, etc. – changed. The fact that the materials coats are made out of have changed from natural to artificial fibres, and that artificial fibres are now a fiftieth of the thickness that they were and so give the fabrics quite different properties; that some materials are waterproof but 'breathable'; that artificial fibres are so much more hardwearing so lending themselves to mixtures of natural and artificial fibres; that materials shrink less; that colours are less likely to come out in the wash; that cars are safer, more comfortable, have much lower petrol consumption than they used to; that domestic fuel has changed from coal to gas and electricity; that gas is burnt in much more efficient central heating boilers so giving more heat for a given level of consumption – all these changes make it almost impossible for price indices to compare like with like.

In the areas such as computers, where quality is increasing fastest, calculations suggest that on a quality-adjusted basis, computer prices have been falling by something like 25 per cent a year (Nelson *et al.* 1994). But the complexity involved in trying to make adequate estimates of the scale of the improvement in the quality of every line of goods in a price index means that price indices are not adequately adjusted for changes in quality. In effect, many improvements in quality which should be set against price rises are ignored. The result is that inflation is overstated and indices of output or of real incomes are deflated by more than they should be. Hence the economic indices give the impression that increases in real living standards are smaller than they actually are.

Although some attempts are made to adjust for quality, Siegal calculated that producer price indices miss about 40 per cent of the changes in the quality of goods and services. This little-known fact is less controversial than might be imagined (Siegal 1994). Siegal also quotes an NBER paper: 'If a poll were taken of professional economists and statisticians, in all probability they would designate – and by a wide majority – the failure of the price indexes to take full account of quality changes as the most important defect in these indexes' (ibid., p. 30). Nordhaus estimated the quality-adjusted changes in the price of light per lumen hour since the beginning of the nineteenth century (Nordhaus 1994). He concluded that conventional price indices would show a 180 per cent rise in the price of light in contrast to the 800 per cent fall which his calculations suggested had actually happened.

The result is not only that we have a mistaken idea of inflation, but every series of figures deflated by a price index is also wrong. If growth averaged about 2 per cent a year over the course of the business cycle, and it was deflated annually by even 1 per cent more than it should have been, then the measure of growth would halve the actual real – quality-adjusted – growth rate. While recognising that in many fields the effect of technical change has been much less dramatic than it has in lighting, Nordhaus nevertheless makes a 'guesstimate' suggesting that increases in real incomes have been many times larger than the conventional indices suggest. Measures of historical trends in the real standard of living are therefore likely to underestimate real progress dramatically.

This suggests that there might be a simple explanation of why at least the rising parts of the curves in figure 3.1 shift to the left with the passage of time: the horizontal distance between the curves could be the improvements in real living standards resulting from unmeasured improvements in the quality of goods and services. How much of what we have called the 'income gearing factor' could be made up of unmeasured qualitative improvements in living standards can be judged by considering whether the curves in figure 3.1 could be amalgamated simply by shifting the more recent curves to the right. It is apparent that the higher part of these curves would have to be shifted further to the right to amalgamate them than the lower parts. But that is plausible. The more a country has departed from traditional goods and traditional methods, the greater is the area of material life which is subject to constant innovation, and the greater is the likely underestimate of its living standards. In other words, the higher the level of development, the more innovation and the greater the missed qualitative changes in goods. Thus accurate figures of GNPpc would lie even further to the right of those shown in figure 3.1 for the richer countries than they would for the poorer ones. Not only would this tend to amalgamate a larger part of the curves, but it would also stretch out the near horizontal part of the curves, bringing them even closer to being truly horizontal.

If increases in GNPpc over time were simply understated, it might be thought that this would not mask a statistical relationship between health and GNPpc: the extent to which societies benefited from qualitative changes in output would be a constant function of their growth rates. If this were so, then understated growth would change the units rather than weaken the correlation between the two. It would tend to make any given increase in income appear more health effective. In technical terms: rather than weakening the correlation coefficient it would increase the size of the regression coefficient. However, it could be argued that the spread of better products does not depend simply on the expenditure which results from the few per cent of income growth. Much nearer to the truth is that, as earlier forms of goods are made obsolete and replaced in the shops by new models and lines, the whole flow of expenditure is applied to the current range of goods, including new goods and ones in which the quality has changed. In other words, the populations of the developed countries benefit from the improvements in the quality of goods in large part independently of the extent to which their incomes have increased, and so independently of their economic growth rates.

British experience provides two powerful demonstrations of the extent to which populations may benefit from technical change, regardless of economic growth rates. Despite Britain's slow economic growth, which has led to its relative decline in relation to other countries, ownership first of televisions, then of videos and most recently of home computers, spread faster in Britain than in almost any other country including much richer ones such as the United States. The spread of new technology and new goods need not be related to economic growth rates. The second example is that over the last ten or fifteen years, although the poorest 10 per cent of the British population has suffered a decline in real incomes and, on average, the bottom 20 per cent has seen no change in their incomes, they have nevertheless dramatically increased their ownership of consumer durables such as freezers, telephones, central heating and videos (Department of Social Security 1993). Although these particular items are not the ones most obviously closely related to health (and we know that at least during the 1980s death rates among the poorest in Britain did not improve (Phillimore *et al.* 1994)), the argument as a whole does show that there are ways in which living standards can improve which are not reflected in the economic indices.

These considerations show that the shifts in the curves in figure 3.1, and the weak correlations between life expectancy and rising GNPpc, should not necessarily be taken as proof that the improvements in mortality are not a product of economic development as properly understood. Indeed, it is hard to think of an explanation for rising life expectancy which is not in some way sustained, enabled or supported by economic development. The evidence for rejecting at least some distant link between rising living standards and increasing life expectancy seems inadequate.

For countries on the horizontal part of the curves in figure 3.1 (which becomes more horizontal in the light of the inadequate quality adjustments), the onus for explaining the upward shift of the life expectancy curve is on the qualitative improvements in living standards which take place over time. If one were to suggest ways in which qualitative change might improve health, one might point to cleaner central heating, which avoids the problems of indoor air pollution and fire hazards associated with open fires; freezers which enable people to eat food with less bacterial contamination; a whole host of developments (including washing machines, electric kettles and disposable nappies) which have made baby and childcare not only easier but also more hygienic and safe; lead-free petrol which reduces environmental pollution; increases in car safety, which have reduced road deaths despite increased car ownership; and the wider provision of phones, which enables families and friends to overcome some of the social dislocation caused by geographical separation (relevant to the powerful influence of social support on health).

Many of these changes sweep the developed world almost simultaneously. Buying and selling in the same world market, among most OECD countries there are relatively small differences in the rate of diffusion of technical changes in the quality of goods. In a sense, the level part of the curve of life expectancy with GNPpc implies that, at least in terms of health, living standards differ only marginally between these countries at any point in time – despite measured differences in GNPpc. Among developed countries a difference of ten or twenty years in the material quality of life would seem to be more important than supposedly large differences in GNPpc at the same point in time.

The more general point which comes out of this is however a distinction between growth as currently measured, and the fruits of worldwide technical change and innovation which can be enjoyed by all developed countries largely independently of differences in their measured growth rates. In essence, we can have improvements in the real standard of living even in the absence of statistical evidence of economic growth. Instead of having more, we have better; and because innovation makes as much difference to methods of production as to the goods produced, we usually have better for much the same price as we paid for that which it replaced. If this picture is true, it provides confirmation of the suggestion that health may be a better guide to trends in the real standard of living than that provided by the various economic indices.

That the main benefits of growth may come through qualitative rather than quantitative improvements in living standards, and that populations may gain from them largely regardless of quantitative growth rates, provides a fundamentally important perspective on the processes by which living standards rise. It is particularly important in relation to the arguments propounded by the environmental movement about the need for 'zero growth' rates. If it were possible to develop price indices which were fully quality-adjusted, the improvements in quality would appear as growth. But it is important to recognise that it may be possible to enjoy the major part (even as much as 90 per cent if we go by the correlations with life expectancy) of the benefits of that growth without necessarily increasing resource use or pollution. The implication is that we need to distinguish between qualitative improvements in living standards and growth which is quantitative, at least in terms of its environmental impact.

So far we have concentrated on explaining the pattern of changes in life expectancy over time shown in figure 3.1. Let us now look more carefully at the changing shape of the cross-sectional relationship between GNPpc and life expectancy. What explanation can be given for its curvature: why among poor countries does life expectancy rise rapidly with increases in GNPpc while among richer countries the relationship levels off and further increases in GNPpc bring little or no improvement in life expectancy? We have seen that the curvature may be partly interpreted as a relationship between given increases in life expectancy and proportional increases in GNPpc – i.e. as a log linear relationship. (I say 'partly' because the rises are rather less than log linear in the developed countries.) However, it should be borne in mind that if the increases in the standard of living are substantially underestimated, particularly at higher levels of development, then the curvature of the relationship with life expectancy would be increased: the countries on the horizontal part of the curve would be spaced out further to the right.

However, there is more to this than the possibility that it may take enormously much larger increases in income to improve health in the developed world than it does in poorer countries. When countries round the corner in the curve relating health to income, they also go through the so-called 'epidemiological transition'. The term is used to demarcate the change from predominantly infectious causes of death, still common in poor countries, to the degenerative diseases which have become the predominant cause of death in richer countries. All the rich developed countries on the nearly horizontal part of the curve went through this transition in their causes of death earlier in the twentieth century. In contrast to the poorer countries on the steeply rising left-hand part of the curve, their death rates are dominated by cardiovascular diseases and cancers rather than by infections.

The epidemiological transition seems to mark a more fundamental turning point in history than is usually recognised. As well as the decline in infections, it also marks a change in the social distribution of a number of important conditions. During the epidemiological transition the so-called 'diseases of affluence' became the diseases of the poor in affluent societies. The most well-known example is coronary heart disease which, in the first half of the twentieth century, was regarded as a businessman's disease but changed its social distribution to become more common in lower social classes. Several other causes of death, including stroke, hypertension, duodenal ulcers, nephritis and nephrosis, and suicide also reversed their social distribution to become more common among the least well-off (Koskinen 1988).

Most revealing, however, was the fact that obesity also changed its social distribution to become more common among the least well-off. This is enormously important. Throughout human history up to this point the rich had been fat and the poor thin. So much so that in many societies obesity was a status symbol and regarded as attractive.

In some preindustrial societies the wives of important men were given especially fattening diets. An ample girth marked people out as belonging to that part of society where there was no shortage of the basic necessities of life. The change in the social distribution of obesity marks a stage in economic development when the vast majority of the population gained regular access to basic necessities. As income levels rose, sugar and other refined foods came to be eaten more by the mass of blue-collar workers and their families than by the rich. (As part of the same process, smoking also moved down the social scale and ceased to be more common in the higher echelons of society.) As some of the less well-off became fat (despite remaining slightly shorter than the rich), obesity ceased to serve as a mark of social distinction. Aesthetic sensibilities changed and, for the first time in history, it became more desirable to be thin than fat. It was during the first half of the twentieth century, under the guidance of Coco Chanel during the interwar years, that the fashion industry began to emphasise slimness.

In terms of the processes of social differentiation, which Bourdieu has shown has such a profound influence on many of our aesthetic judgements, it is interesting to note that, just as slimming became socially desirable when the poor ceased to be hungry, so being sun-tanned started to become desirable when the working population became light-skinned from long hours of indoor factory work (Bourdieu 1984). Earlier, when the poor were sun-tanned agricultural workers, the fashion had of course been to keep the skin as white as possible. Now that rates of obesity are rising dramatically and the poor are characterised as 'couch potatoes', the ideal moves further in the opposite direction and even the icons of beauty of the recent past now look plump.

Another indication that the epidemiological transition marks the attainment of an important threshold in living standards is that the proportion of babies in Britain weighing less than 2,500 grams at birth has remained between 6 and 7 per cent since the 1950s. The fact that the enormous rise in real incomes which has taken place since then has not led to a further reduction suggests that the remaining part of the problem of low birthweights is unlikely to be directly attributable to absolute material living standards.

There are then several important processes which point towards the same interpretation of the flattening part of the curves relating life expectancy to GNPpc in figure 3.1. To summarise, these are the decline in the infectious diseases traditionally associated with poverty, the reversal of social-class gradients in conditions previously associated with wealth – including heart disease and obesity (this latter probably for the first time in recorded history) and lastly, the cessation of the decline in the proportion of low birthweight babies despite rising living standards. Together these suggest that we should probably interpret the levelling off of the curve of rising life expectancy with increasing GNP per capita as the attainment among the majority of the population of a minimum real material standard of living, above which further increases in personal subsistence no longer provide the key to further increases in health. For the bulk of the population, the stranglehold of the absolute standard of living on health has been overcome. Such a transition might have been expected at some stage in the course of economic development. Its appearance as the product of the unprecedentedly rapid and sustained rise in living standards which dates back to at least the middle of the nineteenth century, should not be surprising. If this interpretation is correct, it has fundamental implications for development economics and for thinking on how we should come to terms with global environmental problems.

Having made the point, we now need to recognise a number of important qualifications. First, even in the developed countries which have gone through this transition, there are of course still small *proportions* of the population – but nevertheless large numbers of people – who lack basic necessities including food, shelter and warmth. Although the proportions suffering them are too small to have a substantial influence on overall measures of population health, their numbers are larger than they were, and it is easily within the capacity of developed societies to prevent such conditions entirely. As an indication of how small a proportion of the population in developed countries live with basic material deprivation (rather than the equally serious but quite different effects of relative deprivation which we shall discuss in later chapters), we can turn to the official survey figures showing the ownership of consumer durables among the poorest 20 per cent of the population in Britain (which is now one of the poorer countries in the European Union). Because the survey on which these figures are based has a high non-response rate concentrated particularly among the poorest, they are likely to present too rosy a view of modern poverty, but they do provide a rough guide. In 1990/1 some 98 per cent of the poorest 20 per cent of the population lived in households with a television, 84 per cent had a washing machine, 75 per cent had a freezer (whether or not combined with a fridge) and 97 per cent had a fridge, 72 per cent had a telephone, 72 per cent a central heating system, 59 per cent a video and 47 per cent were in households with a car or van (DSS 1993). While the quality of these goods would of course usually be far below that found in better-off homes, there can be little doubt that levels of consumption even among the badly off are substantially higher than many people recognise when talking about modern poverty. It is against this background that we shall go on in the next chapter to look at the very large differences in death rates and life expectancy which continue to exist between the rich and poor in most developed countries today. A knowledge of current consumption levels is also important when we come to discuss the effects of absolute and relative standards in chapter 5.

Important though they are, none of these qualifications should prevent us recognising the overriding significance to health of the achievement of basic minimum standards for the vast majority of the population. As well as private consumption, we should not forget the role played in these changes by improvements in standards in other spheres of life: in reducing water and air pollution, in the regulation and inspection of working conditions and safety. The health changes which mark the epidemiological transition stand as a testament to the significance of the advance in material living standards across a wide front.

This chapter has developed two major hypotheses to explain the pattern of international increases in life expectancy shown in figure 3.1. First, the succession of new and higher curves may be artefacts of the failure to measure the extent of qualitative improvements in the standard of living. Price indices which are not adequately adjusted for improvements in the quality of goods mean that we have very little idea of the extent of real increases in living standards as they change over time. However, work on the inadequacies of price indices makes it clear that improvements in living standards are substantially underestimated. This means that accurate measures might conceivably resolve the rising parts of the family of curves at different points of time into one curve. One important implication is that life expectancy itself is almost certainly a better guide to living standards than the existing measures of changes over time in real incomes and GNPpc. Second, the curvature of the relationship at each point in time seems likely to reflect sharply diminishing returns to increases in income as economic growth moves countries through the epidemiological transition. During the course of economic growth it is to be expected that a stage will be reached after which improvements in population health are no longer determined primarily by crude increases in the supply of basic necessities. Changes both in the main causes of death and in the social distribution of a number of indicative conditions provide evidence which strongly suggests that the epidemiological transition marks that stage. This has important implications for our understanding of the benefits of economic growth. Not only is it likely that the value of continued economic growth declines after the epidemiological transition, but it may also be true that the most important benefits thereafter come in the form of qualitative improvements in standards rather than from increases in the absolute amount produced. The epidemiological transition seems to contain an important economic message.

In order to discover whether there are ways in which the changing patterns of population health could be related to progress in material living standards, we have been obliged to challenge a number of widely accepted notions about the nature of economic growth and its measures. Despite the difficulties of understanding how the picture of international differences in health and the improvements over time could be plausibly related to economic growth, it is even more difficult to understand how they could *not* be related. Not only is life expectancy higher in more developed countries, but the timing of its historical improvement within each country is clearly associated with economic growth. Because of the all-embracing nature of economic growth (what is *not* related to it?), it is difficult to think of plausible explanations which are not somehow dependent on the growth process. Even factors like educational standards and levels of medical care are intimately related to growth. Indeed, within each country expenditure on medical care tends to rise almost as a constant proportion of GNPpc; though it should be said that the lack of even a suggestion of any international relationship between medical care expenditure and life expectancy is another reason for thinking that medical care is not an important determinant of life expectancy. It is hard to think of candidates for explanations of sustained general improvements in population health which are not in some way enabled or sustained by economic growth. Because one would expect dozens – or more likely hundreds – of factors to contribute, it would seem likely that, on average, progress would be related to the growth process. In that income is a good summary of expanding access to everything that money can buy, one might have thought that health and GNPpc would move closely together. And yet we are left with the perplexing pattern shown in figure 3.1 which we have been trying to explain. Hence the need to see whether there was any way in which our understanding of economic growth could be stretched to fit. The results raise some interesting possibilities but there are components which are far from compelling. Particularly difficult is the problem of putting together the horizontal part of each cross-sectional curve, where the differences between developed countries at any point in time have little or no significance for health, with the evidence that the qualitative changes which take place over time in these countries have great significance. To accept both entails believing that differences between developed countries in the levels of provision of the goods and services available at any point in time matter little, but that the qualitative changes in those goods and services (including knowledge) over time matters very much. Yet, particularly in the light of the probable understatement of the real increase in GNPpc, there can be little doubt that the developed countries are indeed on a horizontal part of the curve that moves upwards over time.

If we are to relate health to material life, we are faced with the suggestion that more of the same in a given time period is less important than qualitative improvements over time. This means believing not only that new knowledge, new technology, new goods and services are important, but also that the rate at which they diffuse in different developed countries is unrelated to exactly where they stand in the scale of affluence among these countries. To some this will sound an unlikely story, but we lack evidence to take the argument further. However, we should not forget the fact that what we are grappling with here is the basic framework for understanding the most important changes going on in health nationally and internationally. Towards the end of chapter 11 we will raise the possibility that health may also have benefited from processes of psychosocial liberalisation which seem to ride piggy-back on economic development. This is one of the few alternative possible sources of the upward movement of the life expectancy curves over time.

Part II

Health inequalities within societies

Chapter 4

The problem of health inequalities

The scale of the health differences within modern societies is surprising. A study which looked at differences in health in the 678 electoral wards of the Northern Region of England found that death rates were four times as high in the poorest 10 per cent of wards as they were in the richest 10 per cent (Phillimore *et al.* 1994). In the United States, a recent study of health in Harlem in New York found that at most ages death rates were higher there than in rural Bangladesh (McCord and Freeman 1990). In Brazil, where income differences are greater than in almost any other country, a study showed that infant mortality rates varied between different areas of the same city from 12 to 90 per 1,000 live births.

Figures like these are not simply a reflection of the scale of poverty in the high mortality areas. The Whitehall study of 17,000 civil servants working in government offices in London found that death rates were three times as high among the most junior office support staff as they were among the most senior administrators (Davey Smith *et al.* 1990). This study population excluded not only the poorest without work but also all manual workers: confined as the study was to employed white-collar workers, these differences occurred among people who would call themselves middle class and who worked together in the same offices.

Numerous studies have shown that the health differences are not confined to differences between the poor and the rest of society, but instead run right across society with every level in the social hierarchy having worse health than the one above it. Data from the Multiple Risk Factor Intervention Trial (MRFIT) in the United States enabled more than 300,000 men to be grouped into twelve income categories according to the median family income of the ZIP code area in which they lived. It showed that incomes and death rates were so closely related across all categories that it made no difference to the positions of eleven out of the twelve groupings whether they were ranked according to ascending income or descending death rates (Davey Smith *et al.* 1992). The gradient in mortality ran across the whole income range from the poorest to the richest (see figure 5.1 on p. 72).

Whatever the difficulties we encountered in the last chapter of understanding the relationship between health and material living standards internationally, there is at least a clear ordering of mortality rates by socioeconomic position within countries. Although research on these health differences within countries has been undertaken almost exclusively to tell us more about health and its determinants, what comes out of it may be more important for what it tells us about society. The fact that in almost any of the rich developed societies people lower down the social scale may have death rates two to four times higher than those nearer the top, seems to give us a fairly blunt message about the nature of modern society. But to understand the message clearly we need to know more about why social position is so closely related to health. Research is providing new insights into how the social structure impinges on us. Nor are the insights confined to issues to do with the way the physical environment affects health. Increasingly it looks as if some of the most important parts of this relationship involve psychosocial pathways: they tell us about the subjective psychological and emotional effects of objective features of the social structure. In this respect, health can tell us about the impact which the social organisation of material life has on human subjectivity. In penetrating the ways in which the social structure has the power of life and death over us, health research reveals some of the most basic links between the individual and the social structure. The 'hard' mortality data and the power of the effects we are trying to understand make it a little easier to penetrate some of the social mirages which normally prevent us understanding the social structure in which we live. As societies are swept along increasingly rapidly by the demands of international economic competitiveness, by the development of electronic technology and the evolution of social institutions at all levels, it becomes increasingly urgent to gain some understanding of the disparate social and economic forces involved.

But before we go any further, it is necessary to summarise a number of essential background issues. We shall start with some problems to do with measures of health, mortality rates and health inequalities. After that we shall go on to the briefest discussions of the reasons why health inequalities cannot be attributed to social mobility, to genetics, to disregarding advice on healthy living, or to differences in medical care. These issues need to be got out of the way before we can return in the following chapters to the fundamental issues of understanding how social and economic processes affect health.

DEATH RATES AND MEASURES OF HEALTH

Death rates are often used – perhaps rather paradoxically – as measures of health because good measures of health and illness do not exist. The problem with illness is not knowing how to count different things: are we to add cases of athlete's foot to cases of arthritis, headaches, chronic bronchitis, hay fever and ulcers? If so, how bad would they have to be to count? If we used pain or disability as a common denominator, how much pain or disability assessed by whom and how often? Because of these almost insurmountable problems, almost the only good data on objectively defined – which of course means doctor-defined – illness comes from Cancer Registries which, in those countries which have them, list all new cases of cancer referred to hospitals. Although various infectious diseases are supposed to be registered by doctors, records are so incomplete that they tell us nothing about incidence or prevalence of infections except in so far as, despite their incompleteness, they indicate trends as epidemics come and go.

Another approach to measuring illness (morbidity) is to forget formal diagnosis and ask people to summarise their own general state of health. A good deal of research uses measures of 'self-assessed health'. You can either ask people a simple question like, 'In the last two weeks has your health been good, fair or poor?' Or you can ask people a list of questions about specific symptoms and then score the answers to give an overall health score. While these measures have important uses, it is often hard to know exactly what they mean. Death rates at least have the advantage of being a fairly clear-cut, accurate and objective measure. Although knowing whether an individual is dead or alive is not a very sensitive measure of health, the variations in age-, sex- and cause-specific death rates from one population or social group to another tells us a good deal more. Differences in death rates are likely to be good indications of differences in disease; and death rates from different causes such as heart disease, bronchitis, cancer and suicide, will give some indication of the scale of such diseases in a society. Their weakness is that they tell us nothing about the prevalence of everyday illnesses and diseases, such as rheumatism, which are not usually life-threatening. Nevertheless, it has been found that there is quite a close relationship between population differences in death rates and differences in the general self-reported measures of illness, which include day-to-day minor ailments (Arber 1987). This suggests that health, though an amorphous concept, does have some coherence across a wide range of diseases and conditions and that differences are measurable.

Death rates express how many deaths there are each year per 1,000 (or 10,000) of the population. Because they increase so dramatically with age, they are usually given for specific age groups – say 15 per 1,000 women in their fifties. Alternatively, you can compare death rates across the whole age range in different populations after taking out the effect of differences in the age structure of the populations. These are age-standardised death rates. Unless you take account of the age composition of the population, places with more old people will appear less healthy than places with a greater number of younger people. Sometimes, to facilitate comparisons between groups, 'standardised mortality ratios' (SMRs) are used. They allow death rates across all ages to be compared between populations after removing the effects of differences in their age structures. (This is calculated by taking the age-specific death rates from the comparison population, applying them to the number of people in each age group in the reference population, and expressing the total number of deaths this would produce in all age groups as a percentage of the number which actually occurred in the reference population.) Measures of illness usually take age into account in much the same way. In this book we shall only discuss differences in death rates and measures of illness after taking account of age.

When told that death rates in one group of people are three or four times as high as in another, it might be imagined that this means that life expectancy must be only a third or a quarter as long. But if we said that people in a rich area of Britain or the United States have a life expectancy of 80 years and death rates in a poor area are four times as high, it would obviously be false to say that life expectancy among the poor is only 20. The arithmetic of how differences in age-standardised death rates affect life expectancy is more complicated than that. The effects are very much smaller because deaths are concentrated mainly in later life where they make less difference to life expectancy. Even among children a fourfold difference in childhood death rates – say, between 2 and 8 deaths per 10,000 children per year – does not have a large impact on overall life expectancy because the death rate is low. The impact would obviously be much bigger if the fourfold difference was between, say, 10 and 40 deaths per 10,000. A calculation made on death rates current in Britain twenty years ago provides a rough guide (OPCS 1978). It shows a linear relationship such that a doubling of age standardised death rates between the ages of 15 and 65 made only a four year difference in life expectancy. Adding in the effect of deaths before age 15 and after age 65 would probably have increased that difference to something like eight years. However, the death rates prevailing now are lower than they were then, so that a doubling of age standardised death rates would make a smaller difference to overall life expectancy at birth.

Perhaps the easiest way of seeing intuitively what the socio-economic differences in death rates mean, is to imagine two people, each with a similar-sized circle of friends and relations – let us say fifty personal contacts – but living in separate rich and poor areas. For every death that occurs among the circle of friends of the person in the rich area, the person in the poor area will know of two, three or even four times as many deaths among his or her circle of friends.

MEASURING HEALTH INEQUALITIES

Saying that death rates in poorer social groups are two, three or four times as high as among richer ones sounds vague. The apparent vagueness is partly a matter of which social groups are being compared, and partly a matter of how accurate the classification of the population into the different groups is. The greater the extremes of wealth and poverty you compare, the bigger the health differences you are likely to find. This is why people living in the poorest 10 per cent of electoral wards in the north of England in the 1980s had death rates four times as high as people in the richest 10 per cent (Phillimore *et al.* 1994).

National figures which classify the economically active population by occupations arranged according to social status typically show twofold or threefold differences in death rates between people in social class I professional occupations (doctors, lawyers, senior government administrators, managers of large companies, etc.) and social class V unskilled manual occupations. However, the occupational information which is used is taken from death certificates based on information supplied by 'next of kin'. It may be difficult to tell whether a 'company director' was a self-employed building worker or a powerful businessman controlling a multi-million pound empire. Similarly, is an 'electrical engineer' a university qualified professional, or an assembly line worker in an electrical components firm? The misclassification of people which results from these difficulties means that the occupational class differences which the calculations yield are inevitably fudged. One indication of how important this fudging may be is shown by the Whitehall study mentioned earlier. The 17,000 civil servants on which it is based were classified by the seniority of their employment grade with the co-operation of the employer. This meant that classification was particularly accurate. Thus, while the national figures find only a twofold difference in death rates between professional and unskilled manual occupations, the Whitehall study found a threefold difference just among office workers.

However, the mortality differences shown in the national statistics are narrower not just because the occupational classification is less accurate. It is probably also partly a reflection of the fact that even within any occupation there are very large differences in things like education and incomes. For instance, rich lawyers as well as poor unemployed lawyers are classified as social class I. A purely occupational classification will be blind to many of the differences that exist within occupational categories. However, in the Whitehall study, in which everyone was a full-time employee working for the same employer, the classification by employment grade would have matched very closely a classification by income and would have come close to a classification by education. In essence, the Registrar General's occupational classes represent much more socioeconomically heterogeneous groupings of people than some other classifications such as the employment grades used in the Whitehall study.

So much for the complexities of measurement. While the reader needs to be aware that they exist, we do not need to dwell on them further.

SOCIAL MOBILITY AND HEALTH

One of the reasons why socioeconomic differences in death rates are regarded as important is that they seem to show the scale of 'excess' – or potentially preventable – mortality in society. The assumption is that if it is possible for some people to have death rates as low as those in upper social groups, then it should be possible to achieve equally low death rates in all groups. Indeed, the amount by which they are higher appears to indicate the number of deaths attributable to something like social and economic deprivation. There was, however, the possibility that the health differences arose from a quite different source. Instead of people having poor health because they were in poorer social and economic conditions, it was suggested that perhaps they were in poorer social and economic conditions because their health was poor. It was suggested, in other words, that people's health was determined largely independently of the conditions in which they lived, and that healthier people were more likely to move up the social pyramid while unhealthy people moved down. The implication was that health inequalities were due to selective social mobility which sorted healthy and unhealthy people into different social classes.

Several large data sets have been used to study this possibility. Data collected from two cohorts of people who have been followed up since birth in 1946 or 1958 are now able to relate early health to subsequent social mobility. Both sets of data found that poor health does effect social mobility but that the size of the effect is too small to account for very much of the overall health differences (Power *et al.* 1990; Wadsworth 1986). Because the people covered by these studies are not yet old enough to show what effects illness in middle age might have on career chances in later life, this part of the issue was tackled using data from the Longitudinal Study (Fox *et al.* 1985). It seemed possible that people who suffered chronic illness later in life might have to give up more demanding jobs and would move down the social scale. For deaths occurring among a 1 per cent sample of the British population at census the Longitudinal Study made it possible to classify deaths according to occupational information given by that person some years earlier. In other words, people could be classified not by what might have been a lower-status occupation during their declining years, but by the occupation they were in some years before death. This too found the effects of illness on social mobility were small. Several other studies, considering both inter- and intragenerational mobility in relation to health, have come to the same conclusions (Lundberg 1991; Blane *et al.* 1993).

A way of getting another angle on this same issue is to look at class differences in mortality among married women or children classified by their husband's or father's occupation. It is reasonably safe to assume that although the 'reference' occupation of husbands or fathers may be affected by their own health, it will be less affected by illness among their wives and children. Thus the large class differences in the health of married women and children when classified by husband's and father's occupation are unlikely to be produced by selective mobility in the job market discriminating between the healthy and the less healthy (Blane *et al.* 1993). The pattern of mortality differences among women classified by their own occupations is much like that for men.

Recently Bartley has shown that the effect of social mobility is likely to make class differences in health smaller rather than larger than they would be without it (Bartley and Plewis, forthcoming 1996). This is because people moving up from lower social classes do not have quite such good health as those born into higher classes. Similarly, people who move down tend to have better health than those who have always been in lower social classes. Both the upward and downward movements therefore tend to dilute the extremes of good and bad health.

The most important contribution which social mobility makes to health differences concerns the upward mobility of taller people who also tend to be healthier (Nystrom Peck 1992). Recent research has shown that, rather than reflecting a genetic advantage, this conjunction of height, health and upward mobility reflects a number of powerful environmental influences in early childhood. We shall discuss this in chapter 10.

HEALTH DIFFERENCES AND GENETICS

The concern with social mobility was essentially a concern that socioeconomic differences in health may be a result of the social fluidity of the population. In the United States however there was a tendency to see similar health differences as if they might be racial in origin. Here, social fixity and genetics were the preferred way of absolving social and economic structures from blame: in essence, opposite strategies serving the same function. Needless to say, research has shown that racial differences in health in the United States are largely accounted for by differences in people's social and economic circumstances.

There have also been suggestions – but no empirical evidence – that there may be genetic differences between social classes which might explain health inequalities (Himsworth 1984). Examination of blood groups across social classes has not produced evidence of genetic differences between them (Kelleher *et al.* 1990). Indeed, one of the few studies to report that there were class differences in blood groups found that the blood group associated with higher intelligence was more common in lower social classes (Mascie-Taylor 1990).

The increased burden of illness from environmental sources would tend to increase the scale of genetic selection for the ability to resist various diseases. Thus it is quite possible that survival of the fittest provides a stronger selective filter for good genes in lower classes where there is more disease. It is certainly argued that wherever easier environmental conditions increase survival chances, it enables the less genetically fit to survive, so harsher conditions and more disease might be expected to select a fitter population. However, the scale of social mobility would ensure that genetic advantages from that source were soon spread throughout the population.

Studies of identical and non-identical twins allow the relative strength of the genetic and environmental components of longevity to be assessed. Hayakawa summarising the results of his own and another study says the results show 'environmental factors to have a strong influence and genetic factors to have a mild influence on the length of human life span' (Hayakawa *et al.* 1992a, p. 184). He also concluded that the low twin concordance rates for the causes of death from which they had died, plus the small differences in the concordance rate for identical and non-identical twins, suggested that environmental influences were the overridingly important determinants of cause of death. (Because identical twins are genetically identical and non-identical twins share – on average – half their genes, the difference in the concordance rates between the two groups can be attributed to the 50 per cent difference in their genetic similarity. Thus the full genetic contribution to the variance is calculated by taking twice the difference between the concordance rates for identical and non-identical twins.)

There are a number of pieces of circumstantial evidence which make it unlikely for there to be a major genetic contribution to health inequalities. First, some of the most important causes of death reversed their social distribution during the middle of the twentieth century: these include coronary heart disease, stroke, hypertension, obesity, duodenal ulcers, nephritis and nephrosis, suicide and lung cancer (Koskinen 1985). There can be little doubt that environmental factors lay behind these changes (Marmot *et al.* 1978a).

As well as reversals in the class differences of some diseases over time, it is also striking that the social gradient in mortality occurs in so many quite different diseases and that the diseases with the steepest gradients vary from one country to another. Thus while coronary heart disease is a major contributor to class differences in mortality in Britain, in France it makes a relatively unimportant contribution (Leclerc *et al.* 1990). France's health inequalities arise primarily from alcohol-related deaths and accidents. In the Scandinavian countries mortality differences from cancers tend to be much less important than they are in France or Britain (Leclerc 1989). If one were to argue that there is a genetic element in socioeconomic success and that it is linked to a lower genetic vulnerability to disease, it would be implausible then to say that it is linked to a reduced vulnerability to different diseases in each of the countries.

The relationship between genetic and environmental contributions to disease is often seriously misunderstood. Too often diseases are regarded as being either genetic or environmental, or some percentage of one and the remainder the rest. These impressions are usually based on data relating the different proportions of people in the population with and without a disease and the different proportions of them with and without various genetic and environmental risk factors. But of course genes and the environment interact. Usually a genetic vulnerability to a disease is a genetic vulnerability to specific environmental risks. We can clarify the difficulty by comparing two diseases. First, imagine a disease that occurs exclusively among a small minority of people with a particular genetic trait. You might say that this disease was virtually 100 per cent genetic. Now think of a disease like chicken-pox or coughs and colds which everyone gets. The fact that all human beings can catch them yet there are other animal species which cannot, means that this disease is also 100 per cent genetic.

In fact the diseases which are said to have a genetic component are merely the sub-category of disease to which genetic differences in the population make some people more vulnerable than others. Yet even among these conditions, the proportion of the disease which seems to be linked to increased genetic vulnerability will vary as exposure to environmental risk factors changes. For example, in developed countries today, much of the variation in height is believed to be an expression of genetic differences. Yet in a poorer society, where malnutrition is common and some people go hungry while others have plenty, the environmental determinants of variations in height would appear much more important than they do in richer countries. Similarly, diseases such as tuberculosis which were said to have an important genetic component, virtually disappeared with environmental change. The environmental circumstances responsible for the disease among both the more and the less genetically susceptible apparently disappeared (though it is now returning). The clear implication is that statements based on cross-sectional evidence (i.e. evidence gathered in a population at one point in time) about genetic components in a disease, may have little relevance to the adoption of a preventive public health strategy.

BEHAVIOURAL RISK FACTORS

Apart from suggested explanations of health inequalities in terms of genetics and selective social mobility, another approach, which incidentally also served to absolve the social structure of responsibility, was to imply that they resulted from differences in people's willingness to adopt a healthy lifestyle. It was suggested that the causes of health differences were to be found in differences in smoking, drinking, diet, exercise and the like. Several large studies have now measured the contribution of factors such as these to differentials in death rates. The fourfold difference in heart disease death rates found between senior and junior staff working in government offices provided a particularly good opportunity to examine the impact of these and other risk factors (Davey Smith et al. 1990). Coronary heart disease is the most important cause of death in which a number of behavioural risk factors are known to be involved. However, the Whitehall study found that all the major known risk factors for heart disease, including those such as blood pressure or short stature which are partly or completely beyond individual control, explained rather little of the gradient in heart disease deaths (Marmot *et al.* 1978b). The shaded part of the columns in figure 4.1 shows the part of the fourfold differences in heart disease which was explained by the major known risk factors. Making allowance for inaccurate measurements of some of the risk factors suggests that the estimate of the proportion of the differences which can be explained should perhaps be increased from just under a third (as shown) to something approaching 40 per cent. If we were to separate out from this 40 per cent just the risk factors which can be at least partially controlled through behaviour change, we might find that something more like a quarter of the differences in heart disease deaths were explained. It has, however, proved very much harder to change behaviour than had once been imagined. Fairly typical are the results of the Multiple Risk Factor Intervention Trial (MRFIT) in the United States, which is the largest trial of behaviour change ever conducted (Multiple Risk Factor Intervention Trial Group 1982). It attempted to change diet, smoking and exercise among white men identified as being in the highest 10 per cent of risk for coronary heart disease. Despite concentrated efforts over six years they only succeeded in making minimal changes. This means that as an approach to prevention, the behavioural route is unlikely to realise anything like the reduction in heart disease which behavioural risk factors appear to contribute. Clearly, behaviour is related to the social context in which people live and is difficult to change in isolation. Indeed, if behaviour was not partly determined by the social environment, there would presumably not be a social class gradient in smoking, in dietary composition or in the amount of leisure-time exercise which people take. In other words, to change behaviour it may be necessary to change more than behaviour.

Despite the unparalleled research effort which has gone into finding the causes of heart disease, most of the modern epidemic is unexplained. Not only do behavioural factors explain only a minority of the social gradient, but they are difficult to alter. As Rose put it, if you are in the lowest risk category for all the behavioural risk factors, your most likely cause of death is still heart disease (Rose 1985).

With the exception of lung cancer and perhaps AIDS, the prospects of tackling health inequalities in other important causes of death through behaviour change are likely to be more limited

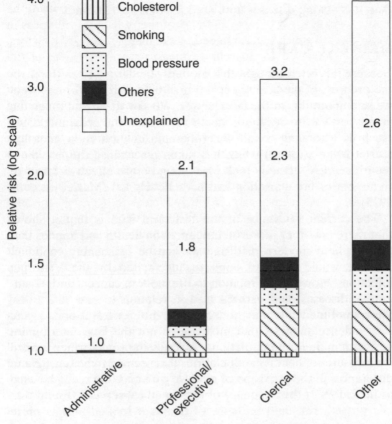

Figure 4.1: Relative risk of death from coronary heart disease according to employment grade, and proportions of differences that can be explained statistically by various risk factors
Note: 'Others' = height, body mass, exercise, glucose tolerance
Source: G. Rose and M. Marmot, Social class and coronary heart disease. *British Heart Journal* 1981: 13–19

than they are for heart disease. This is because in most other causes of death, less is known about behavioural risk factors. Our ignorance of behavioural causes of diseases like stroke or breast or stomach cancer means that the class differences in death rates from these diseases cannot be seen simply as a failure to heed the do's and don'ts of healthy behaviour. That differences in smoking do not dominate the picture is shown by the fact that the social gradient in deaths from diseases related to smoking is no greater than it is among diseases unrelated to smoking (Marmot 1986).

MEDICAL CARE

Because it is often thought that modern standards of health reflect the progress of medical science, it may be worth reaffirming what we said about this in the last chapter. We saw there that much the larger part of the decline in death rates from the great infections (such as whooping cough, flu, tuberculosis, diphtheria, measles, scarlet fever, cholera) which has taken place since the late nineteenth century, actually took place long before effective forms of treatment or immunisation had been developed (McKeown *et al.* 1975).

The current relevance of the historical data is that it shows that there are other powerful influences on health and implies that even without modern medicine we can be reasonably confident that we would not find ourselves decimated by the Victorian infections. However, in relation to the modern cancers and degenerative diseases, and perhaps also in relation to new infections, the role of medicine may now be quite different. But once again, the evidence suggests that medicine is not the key determinant of health in modern populations. A research project which looked for measures of health in populations that seemed to be sensitive to differences in the provision of medical care and that could be used as indicators of the adequacy of local medical services, found that every death rate and measure of health it looked at was more sensitive to variations in socioeconomic conditions than to medical care (Martini *et al.* 1977). Another approach to identifying the benefits of medical care to population health is to define, on the basis of medical expertise, a group of conditions for which good medical treatment ought to be sufficiently successful to prevent almost all deaths. Typically the causes of only 5–15 per cent of all deaths have been categorised as wholly treatable. However, even among these conditions where the influence of medical care ought to be ~~~~~~ 'sed, a review of studies shows that death rates are still ~~~~~ related to social and economic factors than to medical ~~~~~ (Mackenbach *et al.* 1990).

~~~~~ hich provides the most generous assessment of the ~~~~~ ical care, involved the use of medically informed ~~~~~ e benefits provided by each of the main areas of

medical services, including screening, immunisation and the main areas of treatment. Despite estimating rather than measuring benefits, it concluded that the total benefits of all existing forms of medical prevention and treatment added at most five years to the life expectancy of Americans (Bunker *et al.* 1994). Setting this alongside the total gain of close to twenty-five years in American life expectancy during the twentieth century, it suggests that medicine has contributed no more than 20 per cent of it.

The smallness of any influence which medical care may have on population health is not however a reason for thinking it is ineffective. An army medical corps may do invaluable work on battle wounds and yet never be an important determinant of the number of casualties in a battle. In terms of civilian health, the battlefield is the social and economic circumstances in which we live. Much more important than the small differences medicine can make in survival from cancers and heart disease are differences in the incidence of these diseases. In many cases the scope for medical intervention is extremely limited: the first symptom of heart disease is often sudden death. Essentially it is the nature of social and economic life rather than medical services which determines the health of populations: the role of medicine is to pick up the pieces. However, the importance even of that role should not be underestimated. The quality of life, particularly of old people, is greatly enhanced by a whole range of routine procedures such as cataract operations, hernia repairs, pain relief, hip replacement and the removal of varicose veins.

Given the relatively small contribution of medical services to the health of the population as a whole, it is not surprising that differences in medical care make a negligible difference to health inequalities. In countries where medical care is not provided free to all, research workers have shown that it makes little difference to include access to medical care as a control variable in analyses of health inequalities (Haan *et al.* 1987). Work on socioeconomic differences in survival after cancer and heart disease suggests that the survival differences are not primarily the result of differences in treatment (Leon and Wilkinson 1989). Under the National Health Service in Britain, at least one piece of research has suggested that the distribution of medical care may favour the poor, even after allowing for their increased frequency of ill-health (O'Donnell *et al.* 1989).

HEALTH INEQUALITIES ARE VARIABLE

Before the spate of recent research on health inequalities, and indeed before it was clear that socioeconomic differences in health were not reducible to differences in medical care, behavioural choices, social mobility or genetics, it seemed quite likely that they arose from features of society that were too deeply embedded in the fundamental social and economic inequalities of modern life to change. Although governments may be all-powerful in constitutional theory, in practice they often have rather little room for manoeuvre: even if they have the political will, facing down powerful vested interests without the support of a politically active population is often dangerous. But the impression that different governments make only a superficial impact on the social and economic structure, while health inequalities have their roots in much deeper and more permanent features, is at least partly contradicted by the evidence. Our increased ability to measure changes in health inequalities over time, and to make comparisons from one country to another, shows that they are variable. Health inequalities in Scandinavian countries tend to be smaller than they are for instance in Britain and a number of other countries. In countries such as the United States, Britain and France, health inequalities have widened during recent decades, while in others, such as Japan, they seem to have been stable or diminishing. This evidence of variability over time and between countries is important: it shows that the extent of health inequalities is not fixed but is sensitive to the kind of differences which already exist between countries and occur from time to time in the developed world. They show that large health inequalities are not a fact of modern life that we have to live with.

That health inequalities can widen despite growing prosperity is important. Instead of diminishing under the impact of postwar prosperity, health inequalities in Britain have widened almost continuously since the middle of the twentieth century. The evidence for this comes from the official figures on occupational mortality produced every ten years. They have shown widening differences during each decade since the 1951 census. In the context of growing prosperity during the postwar decades, the widening seemed counter-intuitive and there was a tendency to doubt the figures. It was suggested that it was a false impression created by the changing class distribution of the population as the proportion of people in the lower manual occupational classes dwindled and the numbers in the higher white-collar occupations increased. It was forgotten that, in terms of the size of the gap, any argument about the effect of the more extreme death rates obtained from a shrinking – and therefore perhaps more socioeconomically extreme – group at the bottom would be offset by the less extreme rates obtained from the growing group at the top. It was also suggested that the decennial revisions to the class classification of occupations invalidated comparisons over time. These problems were resolved by an American researcher using the *slope index of inequality* which, instead of just comparing the extreme social classes, measured the extent of mortality inequality across the whole population while weighting each class by the proportion of the population in it (Pamuk 1985). Pamuk dealt with the problem of revisions in the classification of occupations by selecting those occupations which she could identify consistently all the way through the period covered by her comparisons. She showed results using the class allocations of the occupations fixed as they were at the beginning of the period, fixed as they were at the end of the period, and then varying as the class allocations changed during the period. Regardless of the methods, the results gave a robust picture of narrowing health inequalities before the middle of the century and a widening gap thereafter.

Another criticism of the original official figures for England and Wales was that making up death rates by matching the occupations given on death certificates by 'next of kin' with the population numbers in each occupation taken from the census might be unreliable. There were, for instance, suggestions that next of kin have a tendency to 'promote the dead'. The self-employed might, for instance, be reported by relatives as company directors. (Interestingly, Dore says that occasionally Japanese firms will promote people posthumously as a tribute to them (Dore 1973).) It was partly to overcome difficulties of the former kind that the OPCS Longitudinal Study was started. Instead of using the occupations given on death certificates, it was able to relate each death back to the occupation given by the deceased at the last census. Once again the results suggested that the official figures had not been misleading.

We have now seen that health inequalities cannot be understood in terms of biased measurements, selective social mobility, genetic differences, inequalities in medical care or health-related behaviour. Nor should it be thought that each contributes a small part which when added together explains a large part of the picture. First, inaccurate social classification makes health differences look smaller than they really are. Second, while there is health-related social mobility, there are reasons for thinking that the effect of all social mobility combined tends to diminish the differences (Bartley and Plewis, forthcoming 1996). Third, there is no evidence that there is any significant genetic contribution and quite a lot of circumstantial evidence to suggest that there is not. Fourth, not only is the overall effect of medical care on population health small enough to be hard to measure but, at least in Britain, the poor use more medical services than the better-off. Whether this is enough to make up for their greater need is the subject of some academic controversy – which presumably means there is not an enormous mismatch. Lastly, while health-related behaviour does account for a significant minority of the overall differences, and a majority in lung cancer and AIDS, two things should be remembered: first, that differences in death rates from the major causes of death unrelated to obvious behavioural risk factors are still large, and second that the social patterning of behavioural risk factors shows that they are also influenced by the socioeconomic environment.

By this process of elimination we arrive at the conclusion that the differences in health associated with differences in socioeconomic status have to be explained very largely in terms of those socioeconomic differences. But this conclusion does not rest simply on the elimination of other possible explanations. In subsequent chapters we shall see positive evidence of what appear to be causal relationships between health and particular features of socioeconomic life. Disentangling the important causal pathways from the web of associations is difficult because almost all measures of health are associated with almost all measures of socioeconomic status. Without intending to make any claims to direct causality, researchers have shown steep mortality gradients related to variables taken from the census like car ownership and whether people own or rent their housing. Using these and occupational class, it is possible to construct a matrix of increasing deprivation, starting with upper-class people with cars living in their own homes, and ending up with people in unskilled manual occupations without a car who live in rented accommodation. Each step down this hierarchy is associated with a step up in death rates (Goldblatt 1990).

A very wide range of causes of death is involved in health inequalities. Sixty-five of the 78 most important causes of death among men are more common in manual than non-manual occupations, and 62 of the top 82 among women (Townsend *et al*. 1988). This means that a disease-by-disease approach to tackling socioeconomic influences in health is unlikely to be successful. Dealing with individual risk factors for individual causes of death is an approach to prevention which has severe limitations. Rose calculated that in order for seat belts to save the life of one car crash victim '399 [people] would have worn a seat belt everyday for 40 years without benefit to their survival' (Rose 1981). Similarly, using data from the Framingham study, he calculated the effect of a low cholesterol diet on individual risks of heart attack. If men were to modify their diet enough to reduce their cholesterol levels by 10 per cent up to the age of 55, 98 per cent of them would have to eat differently every day for forty years without having prevented a heart attack by doing so. These calculations do not come from someone taking unrepresentative figures to rubbish preventive policies. They are instead the conclusions based on the best data available drawn by a highly respected academic who devoted much of his life to preventive health. If the pay-offs to individuals are so small even for the preventive measures which are regarded as most important, what hope is there for less important risk factors in less important causes of death? Once again we are faced with the need to develop preventive policies from a more social and structural view of the determinants of health.

Chapter 5

Income distribution and health

One of the most important issues arising from the last two chapters is the contrast between them. We saw in chapter 3 that the differences in income and health between developed countries are, at best, only very weakly related; yet in chapter 4 we saw that within developed countries they are almost always very closely related.

Cross-sectional data showing the contrast between the fit within countries and the lack of a fit between them is illustrated in figures 5.1 and 5.2. Figure 5.1 shows American data covering some 300,000 white men in the Multiple Risk Factor Intervention Trial (MRFIT). Death rates are related to the average household incomes of the US zip code areas in which they lived. The regularity with which death rates decline with increasing income is striking. This regular gradient turns up again and again. It was illustrated in another form in figure 4.1, on p. 65, which used British data from the 17,000 strong Whitehall study of civil servants. As we saw in the last chapter, close relationships exist between almost any measure of health and socioeconomic status. The overall mortality gradient among the civil servants is steeper than in the US data probably because they are more accurately classified by socioeconomic status. The Whitehall study's classification was a classification by individual socioeconomic status undertaken with the employer's co-operation and so is extremely accurate. To a large extent differences in occupational grade, level of education and income would have been closely related. On the other hand, MRFIT data using average incomes of the area of residence would classify rich people living in poor areas as poor and vice versa. This will lead to some fudging of the mortality differences.

Figure 5.2 shows that among the developed market economies belonging to the OECD there is no similarly regular gradient in

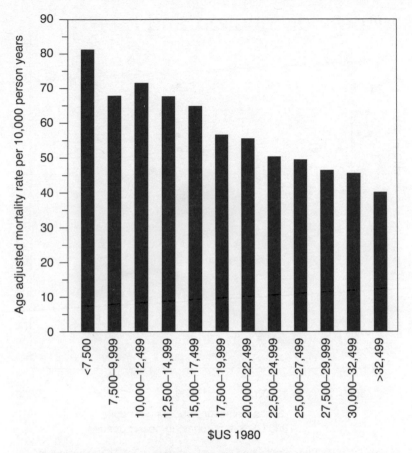

Figure 5.1: Income and mortality among white US men
Source: MRFIT data from G. Davey Smith, J.D. Neaton and J. Stamler,
Socioeconomic differentials in mortality risk among 305,099 white men

average life expectancy related to GNPpc. For what the data on changes over time are worth, the correlation between changes in GNPpc and life expectancy in the same group of countries during the twenty years 1970–90 confirms that this relationship is no closer than the cross-sectional one shown.

How then can we resolve the apparent paradox that income is closely associated with health within countries but not between them? The explanation is not a matter of some artifactual distortion of the data. The weaknesses in the GNP data which we discussed in chapter 3 mean only that the horizontal axis should perhaps

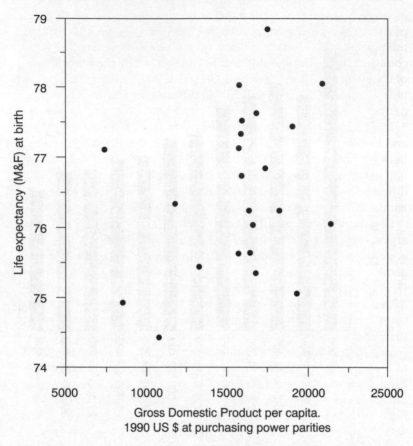

Figure 5.2: GDP per capita and life expectancy in OECD countries in 1990

be stretched out further to the right so that the differences in GNPpc between countries are progressively increased. Such a change would do nothing to improve the ordering of countries or to produce anything like the smooth gradient seen in figure 5.1.

As the points in figure 5.2 are whole countries, there is no possibility that the lack of a clear gradient has something to do with problems of sampling error or random variation. Nor could it be that the international data are more influenced by national differences in culture than by differences in the standard of living. The GNP figures used are converted at purchasing power parities rather than at the rather arbitrary currency exchange rates. This means that they give a more accurate reflection at least of comparative differences in purchasing power. If a much stronger relationship was merely hidden by cultural differences between countries, then that should have been revealed by the correlations of changes over time between 1970 and 1990 (see figure 3.2, p. 37) unless cultures changed radically in different directions during the period.

It is difficult to explain away the contrasting relationships within and between countries as in some way artefactual. The mismatch between the regular gradient shown in figure 5.1 and the lack of one in figure 5.2 has to be taken seriously. It strongly implies that differences in living standards mean something quite different within and between countries.

Fortunately this paradox can be quite easily resolved. It was argued in chapter 3 that among the developed countries which have gone beyond the threshold standard of living marked by the epidemiological transition (see p. 44), further increases in measured GNPpc make little difference to health. This was shown by the flattening of the curves in figure 3.1. (If valid, the suggestion that the data did not adequately take into account the improvements in the quality of goods would only have served to emphasise this flattening.) However, within countries the differences in the standard of living establish a social ordering of the population. What affects health is no longer the differences in absolute material standards, but social position within societies. The paradox would be resolved if it were the health effects of relative income which we could see within countries. On that basis, what matters would not be whether you have a larger or smaller house or car in itself, but what these and similar differences mean socially and what they make you feel about yourself and the world around you.

That we are indeed dealing with the effects of relative rather than absolute income within countries can be clearly demonstrated. Although we cannot look at people's income and health and distinguish between the effects of absolute and relative income individually, we can distinguish between countries with more or less relative poverty. Countries in which the income differences between rich and poor are larger (meaning more or deeper relative poverty) tend to have worse health than countries in which the differences are smaller. It is, as we shall see, the most egalitarian rather than the richest developed countries which have the best health.

Figure 5.3 shows the relationship between the share of total personal income received by the least well-off 70 per cent of families (which, because poorer households tend to contain fewer people than richer ones, amounts to the least well-off 50 per cent or so of the population) and average life expectancy. Life expectancy in countries like Sweden and Norway, where the poorest 70 per cent of households received a larger share of income than elsewhere, is higher than it is in countries like the former West Germany and the United States which were less egalitarian.

Looking at changes in the scale of income differences over time reveals the same relationship. Figure 5.4 uses data from a study of changes in relative poverty between 1975 and 1985. Relative

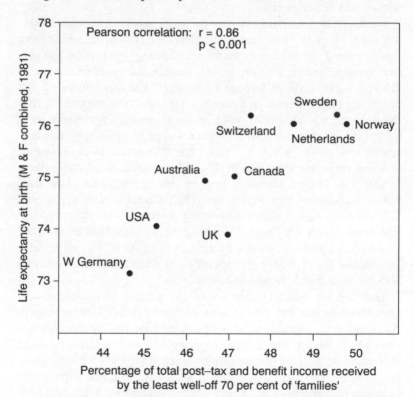

Figure 5.3: The cross-sectional relationship between income distribution and life expectancy (M&F) at birth in developed countries, *c*. 1981
Source: Data from J.A. Bishop, J.P. Formby and W.J. Smith, International comparisons of income inequality: Luxembourg Income Study, 1989: Working paper 26.

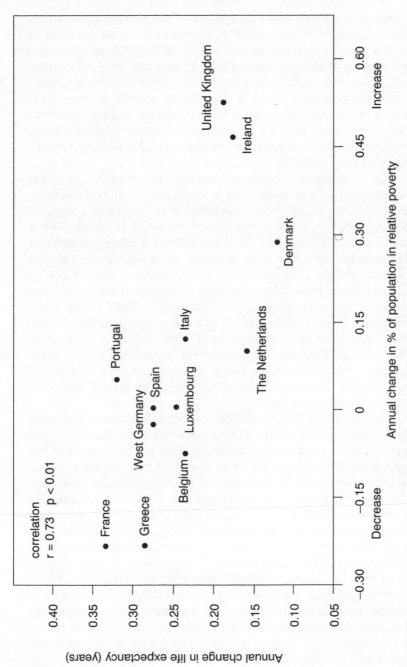

Figure 5.4: The annual rate of change of life expectancy in twelve European Community countries and the rate of change in the percentage of the population in relative poverty, 1975–85
Source: Data from M. O'Higgins and S.P. Jenkins, Poverty in the EC. In: R. Teekens, B.M.S. van Praag (eds) *Analysing poverty in the European Community,* Luxembourg, EUROSTAT, 1990

poverty was defined as the proportion of the population receiving less than half the average income. It shows that those countries of the European Union that diminished the proportion of their population living in relative poverty (e.g. France and Greece) enjoyed faster increases in life expectancy than those in which relative poverty increased. (Changes in life expectancy and in the proportion of the population living in relative poverty during the period 1975–85 are expressed at annual rates. Because of problems in the mortality data, the figures for Portugal cover the years 1981–85 only (Wilkinson 1995)).

The relationship between income distribution and life expectancy was first discovered in data from both rich and poor countries. Among a group of some fifty-six rich and poor countries, Rodgers showed that life expectancy was related to both GNPpc and to income distribution (Rodgers 1979). Statistically significant relationships have now been reported by at least eight different research groups using some ten separate sets of data drawn at different dates, from different groups of developed and developing countries on cross-sectional and time series bases (Flegg 1982; Wilkinson 1986, 1992, 1994b; Le Grand 1987; Waldmann 1992; Wennemo 1993; Kaplan, G. A. *et al.* 1996; Kennedy, B. P. *et al.* 1996). While Flegg looked exclusively at developing countries, Rodgers and Waldmann looked at countries at various stages of development. The others were all concerned exclusively with data from developed countries.

In his analysis of data from some seventy rich and poor countries, Waldmann found that if the absolute incomes of the poorest 20 per cent in each society are held constant, rises in the incomes of the top 5 per cent are associated with *rises* in infant mortality. Given that one might have expected that rises in the incomes of the richest would, other things being held equal, have led to a reduction in their infant mortality, this is a particularly powerful demonstration of the importance of relative income. Also working on infant mortality, Wennemo found a close cross-sectional association between it and the extent of relative poverty in developed countries. Among a group of seventeen developed countries Le Grand found that average age of death was related to income distribution. As well as holding internationally, working quite separately, Kaplan and Kennedy have both shown that the relationship also holds within the United States. The American states with wider economic differences also have higher mortality rates. The raw data – which were kindly supplied by Kaplan and Lynch – are shown in figure 5.5 (Kaplan *et al.* 1996). It shows a correlation of 0.62 (P < 0.001) between the age-adjusted death rate from all causes combined and the percentage share of household income received by the least well-off 50 per cent of the population. The relationship remains highly significant even after controlling for average incomes, absolute poverty, racial differences and smoking (Kaplan *et al.* 1996; Kennedy *et al.* 1996). Kaplan found in addition that the states with wider income differences showed slower improvements in mortality between 1980 and 1990. Ben Shlomo working on data covering small areas in Britain also found a statistically significant tendency for areas with more equality to have lower mortality

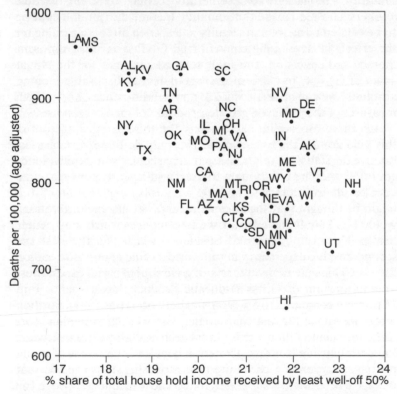

Figure 5.5: The relationship between income distribution and mortality among fifty states of the USA in 1990
Sources: Data calculated from US Census and National Centre for Health Statistics by Kaplan, Pamuk, Lynch, Cohen and Balfour (1996), who kindly provided it for publication here

rates, even after controlling for average deprivation levels in each area (Ben Shlomo *et al.* 1996).

As well as the work on mortality rates, Steckel reported a relationship between average height (which is closely related to health) and income distribution (Steckel 1983, 1994). Comparing the relative power of the relationships of income distribution and per capita economic growth to height, Steckel says that the effect on adult height of a doubling of per capita income could be offset by a modest rise of 0.066 in the Gini coefficient of income inequality.

Given that the relationship between health and income distribution exists, how confident can we be of its meaning? Could it be a spurious reflection of some other more important underlying relationship? The various control variables which different research workers have used make this unlikely. Income distribution appears to be related to national mortality rates, even after controlling for the effects in developing countries of: GNPpc, fertility, maternal literacy and education; and in developed countries for the effects again of GNPpc, but also of average personal disposable income, absolute levels of poverty, smoking, racial differences, and various measures of the public or private provision of medical services.

But there are additional reasons for thinking that factors of this kind are not the explanation. Not only do these variables not remove the statistical relationship but, particularly in the developed countries, they are not thought to exert a sufficiently powerful influence on life expectancy to provide a plausible explanation of it. It might be thought that societies with narrower income differentials would be likely to have better welfare services which may benefit health. However, Japan and Sweden – which had the best and second-best life expectancy in the world – came at opposite ends of the OECD league table in terms of government social expenditure as a proportion of Gross Domestic Product: Japan spends only 15 per cent compared to Sweden's 40 per cent (Hills 1994). Furthermore, we saw in the last chapter that factors such as medical care make too small a difference to population mortality rates to account for a relationship like this. The same goes for other areas of public provision. Even if we ignore the results of using statistical controls, there are no obvious candidates for factors which might prove this relationship to be spurious.

It seems very unlikely that there is a sufficiently powerful unknown variable. If a statistical association were to be explained away as a reflection of a more powerful underlying relationship, the underlying relationship would need to be stronger than the spurious relationship to which it gives rise. This means that it would be much easier to explain away a weak relationship as spurious than to explain away a relationship as strong as the one we are dealing with here.

An important additional problem in treating this relationship as a product of some underlying variable is the number of situations in which it would have to intervene to the same effect. First, it would have to work not only among developed countries, but also in the very different conditions found in developing countries. Second, it would have to explain the cross-sectional evidence as well as that from data dealing with changes over time. Third, as well as the international association between income distribution and national mortality rates, it would have to explain relationships between the amount of inequality and mortality within areas of the same country. The two reports that mortality in fifty states of the United States is related to the amount of income inequality within them were tightly controlled for a number of potential confounders (Kaplan, G. A. *et al.* 1996; Kennedy, B. P. *et al.* 1996). The association was also found when looking at changes over time (Kaplan, G. A. *et al.* 1996). Also within a country there is the cross-sectional association reported by Ben Shlomo using British small area data (Ben Shlomo *et al.* 1996). In this case the effects, though statistically significant, were fairly weak – probably because many of the important social structures which define our social position are not confined to small areas but involve wider processes of social comparison. Even if it were thought that features of public policy in more egalitarian countries might explain the international relationship between income equality and health, they could not explain such a relationship within countries (except perhaps by reference to local differences in public policy).

The evidence of a relationship between economic equality and population mortality rates is much too strong to be dismissed, and it is found on too many different bases for it to be an expression of some intervening variable. Indeed, income has such a powerful direct effect on so many facets of people's lives, that a direct effect on health is very much more plausible than other explanations.

But even given a 'real' relationship, some might question which way round it works. Could there be a process of 'reverse causality' by which health might be affecting income distribution? If the arrow of causality pointed in that direction, we would be obliged to say that health is one of the most important determinants of income distribution. Not only does this run counter to economic theory, but it flies in the face of commonsense notions of the influence on income distribution of employment and unemployment, profits, taxes and benefits. In addition, the data on class differences in mortality have been thoroughly examined for the effects of reverse causality – that is to say, for the possibility that health inequalities appear because people with good health move up the social scale while those with poor health move down (see p. 59). Although this happens to a small extent, it does not account for the bulk of health inequalities. If that were true of class differences in health, which are measured among the economically active population of working age where health would be most likely to effect occupational mobility, how much more true must it be of national life expectancy across all age groups, which includes economically inactive children and old people among whom changes in health would have little or no effect on income? But any reverse causality could not simply be a relationship between individual selective social mobility (or income mobility) and health: it would have to be a relationship between societal levels of health – however distributed – and societal income inequality.

At one time it seemed plausible that income distribution would affect mortality in quite different ways in rich and poor countries. In poorer countries where increases in the absolute standard of living are still important, it seemed likely that narrower income differences might mean that a smaller proportion of GNPpc was being spent on luxuries which would be of little benefit to health, while more would be spent on health-producing necessities. Presumably the higher the proportion of consumer expenditure which is spent on bread for the many rather than yachts and grand houses for the few, the better the population's health will be. In this way, the health benefits of narrower income differences would result less from the purely social effects of the income differences themselves, than from the effects of the higher absolute levels of consumption among the poor. In developed countries, where the GNPpc data suggest that absolute living standards are well above critical levels, the health effects of narrower income differences seem (as we shall see in chapter 8) much more likely to result from the psychosocial effect of inequality, or relative poverty *per se*.

Although it seemed a little awkward to have quite different explanations for what seemed to be the same phenomenon in developed and less developed countries, it was not until Waldmann published his paper that it became clear that this duality could not be sustained. To recap, in his analysis of some seventy countries Waldmann found – rather to his own surprise – that if you held the incomes of the poorest 20 per cent of the population constant in absolute terms (controlling statistically), then the higher the incomes of the richest 5 per cent were, the higher also were the infant mortality rates. Any effect of real incomes on material standards would lead one to expect that if the incomes of the poorest 20 per cent were held constant, any rise in the absolute incomes of the richest 5 per cent would – if anything – lead to slightly lower infant mortality as the children of the rich would do marginally better. To find that the opposite is the case is important; it suggests that there is a genuinely social effect of income inequality among poorer as well as richer countries for which we must seek a unified understanding.

We saw in chapter 3 that during the epidemiological transition health ceases to be so affected by the absolute standard of living. I argued (elsewhere) that there was a transition from health being affected by absolute standards to it being affected by relative standards (Wilkinson 1994a). However, it would be more accurate to say that it is affected by relative standards both before and after the transition, but becomes less affected by absolute standards after the epidemiological transition. We shall look at the likely mechanisms by which reduced income inequality improves health in chapters 8, 9 and 10.

Perhaps the most striking example of the way narrowing income differences can improve health – or rather life expectancy – comes from Japan. The earliest set of income distribution figures which are broadly comparable internationally are for 1970 and include Japan (Sawyer 1976). The relationship between income distribution and life expectancy at that date is shown for the countries covered by that data in figure 5.6. (Though it uses different measures and data from a different source, this figure looks much like figure 5.3. It is included here only for the sake of its Japanese data.) The measure of income distribution used in figure 5.6 is the Gini coefficient, which measures inequality across the whole population rather than by just comparing the rich and poor. Its value varies between 0, which would mean everyone had the same income, and 1, which would mean all income went to one individual and no one else would have any. This means that a value of 0.4

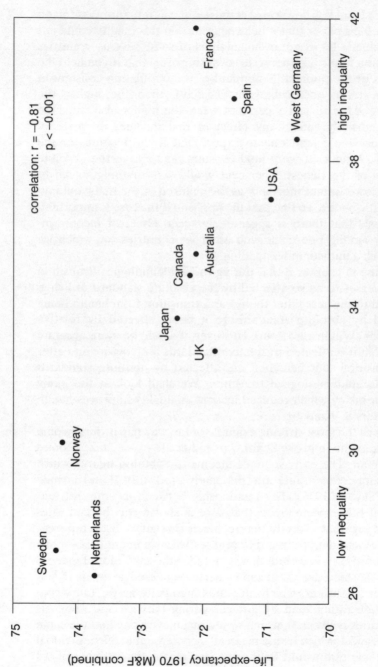

Figure 5.6: Life expectancy (M&F) and Gini coefficients of post-tax income inequality (standardised for household size)
Sources: Data from M. Sawyer, Income distribution in OECD countries, OECD Economic Outlook, Occasional Studies, 1976, 3–36, Table 11; and World Bank

(to the right on the horizontal axis) represents greater inequality than 0.3. Japan appears in the middle of the field with income distribution and life expectancy much like Britain's at that date. However, almost twenty years later a paper appeared in the *British Medical Journal* pointing out that by 1989 life expectancy in Japan had become the highest in the world (Marmot and Davey Smith 1989). It also mentioned that at the same time Japan had achieved the narrowest income differences of any country reporting to the World Bank (that almost certainly means of any developed market economy). The paper's authors say that the improvement in Japanese life expectancy between 1970 and 1986 is equivalent to the gain in life expectancy in Britain which would follow from the elimination of all deaths from heart disease and most cancers. They go through the possible sources of this remarkable achievement, looking for changes in Japanese diet, smoking and other behavioural factors affecting health, in health services and preventative health policies. None of these provides a plausible explanation. Although Japanese diets are healthier than many Western diets, they did not change during this period in ways that might explain the health improvement. Although Japanese economic growth has of course been rapid, not only have we seen that increases in GNPpc are not so important in the developed world but, on the basis of purchasing power parities used to compare living standards more accurately, Japanese GNPpc was only 15 per cent higher than the British in 1990 – still considerably less than the United States and a number of Western European countries.

It is not just since 1970 that the Japanese experience has testified to the health importance of narrowing income distribution. There is also some fragmentary data which shows an earlier association between narrowing income differences and the rapid improvements in life expectancy in Japan (Wilkinson 1992).

Narrower differences in income may be associated with improvements in population health in two mutually compatible, but different, ways. First, in societies with narrower income differences it might be that the quality of the social fabric somehow means that health is better in all sections of society – from top to bottom. Second, average health and life expectancy might increase or decrease primarily as the health of poorer people improves or deteriorates with changes in the scale of their relative poverty. Do narrower income differences lead to a differential improvement in health among the least well-off, so narrowing health inequalities, or do they act primarily by improving the health of the whole population while having less effect on health differences? Because these two possibilities are not mutually incompatible, one might expect both patterns to be operating. The question would then become a matter of the relative importance of each.

One approach to answering the question would seem to be through international comparisons. Although different countries use different social class classifications which increases the difficulty of comparing health inequalities internationally, some Swedish researchers have enabled us to make fairly accurate comparisons of social class differences in mortality between Sweden and England and Wales (Vagero and Lundberg 1989; Leon *et al*. 1992). A large number of Swedish deaths were reclassified according to the British social class classification system. The comparison which this allows is particularly useful because income distribution is much more egalitarian in Sweden than in England and Wales. Figures 5.7 and 5.8 show the social class gradient in mortality for infants and adult males aged 20–64 years. (Unfortunately figures for women were not given.) In both cases the class gradient is much less steep and less consistent in Sweden than it is in England and Wales. However, as well as the class gradients being shallower, we can also see that the groups with the worst mortality in Sweden have lower mortality rates than the best (social class I) in England and Wales. So although England and Wales have bigger income differences and bigger mortality differences than Sweden, the apparent mortality improvement in Sweden compared to England and Wales is not just confined to the most deprived social groups. If – for the sake of argument – narrower income differences were all that was needed to get from the mortality position of England and Wales to that of Sweden, it looks as if everyone would benefit, but that the relatively poor would benefit most.

However, all may not be quite what it seems. People in social class I are not uniformly prosperous. Because this is a purely occupational classification, solicitors and doctors would still go down as social class I even if they were unemployed. In addition, there are large differentials in earnings within each occupation. Thus social class I death rates in Sweden might be lower than in England and Wales not because the benefits of narrower income differentials extend even to the rich, but because even social class I includes a small proportion of poor people who are perhaps less poor where income differences are narrower.

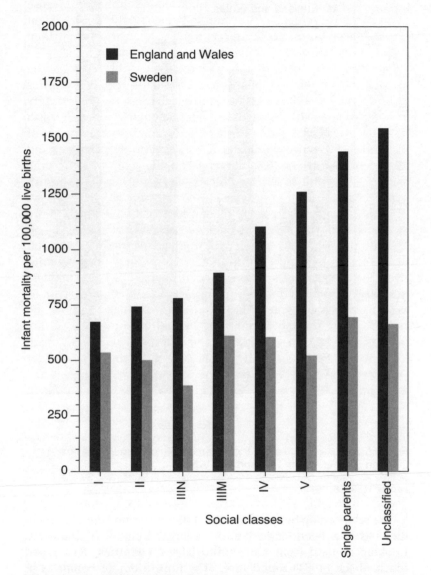

Figure 5.7: Social class differences in infant mortality in Sweden compared with England and Wales
Source: Leon *et al*. 1992

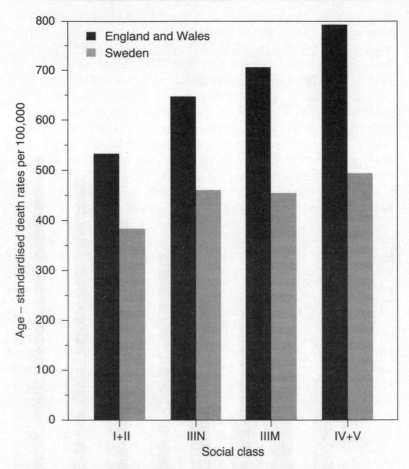

Figure 5.8: Social class differences in mortality of men 20–64 years:
Sweden compared with England and Wales
Source: D. Vagero, O. Lundberg. Health inequalities in Britain and Sweden.
Lancet 11: 35–6. 1989.

The relationship between income differences and health inequalities has now been studied across a larger number of countries.
Looking at data from nine industrialised countries, Kunst and
Mackenbach (1994) found that, 'The rank order of countries in
terms of income inequalities strongly corresponds to their rank
order in terms of inequalities in mortality.' Since then van
Doorslaer *et al.* have reported that differences in self-reported
illness were greatest in countries whose income differences were

greatest (van Doorslaer *et al.* 1996). The relationship between measures of inequality in income and in illness was very close: across the USA and the eight European countries for which they had data, the correlation coefficient was 0.87. The methods used in each study were quite different. Kunst and Mackenbach classified people according to occupation in one of their studies and by education in another, and they concluded that occupational and educational differences in mortality were greater in countries where income differences were greater. In contrast, van Doorslaer *et al.* used data from surveys giving details of incomes and self-reported health for the same individuals.

Another indication of whether narrower income differences benefit the health of the whole population or only that of the least well-off might be to establish the proportion of the population whose income share is most closely related to average life expectancy. Is average life expectancy most closely related to the share of income going to just the bottom 10 or 20 per cent of the population, or is the share received by the bottom 50, 60 or even 70 per cent more closely related to national standards of health?

The first time I looked at this question the results seemed fairly clear. Using data for the countries shown in figure 5.3 and correlating life expectancy in each country with the share of income received by the bottom 10, 20, 30 and so on up to 90 per cent, I found that the relationship became gradually stronger until it reached its maximum around the share going to the bottom 60 or 70 per cent, after which it weakened again (Wilkinson 1992). Hence figure 5.3 shows life expectancy plotted against the share of income received by the least well-off 70 per cent. However, this was a percentage of households – not of population. As poorer households tend to contain fewer people than richer ones (the effects of poor old people living alone or in couples outweighs the effects of poor families with lots of children), the bottom 60 to 70 per cent of families contain something like 50 per cent of the population. So the answer seemed to be that average life expectancy was related most closely to the relative incomes of the least well-off half of the population.

More recent analysis of data which has since become available for a larger number of developed countries has however complicated this picture. Instead of the bottom 50 per cent, the relationship was closest with the income share of the poorest 30 per cent. Which figure is the better guide is hard to say, and indeed the relationship may be expected to differ according to how relatively poor the poor are in each country. In addition there are problems of data quality. It became clear when analysing the later data that the figures from some countries are badly distorted by people who do not respond to surveys of personal income. All the data come from official surveys of households in which people are asked questions about their income. In a few of these surveys, answers are only obtained from some 50 or 60 per cent of the sampled households, and most are below 75 per cent. Unfortunately the non-responders tend to be concentrated among the poor and, to a lesser extent, the rich (Wolf, W. 1988; Redpath 1986). This means that the poor and the rich are underrepresented in surveys with low response rates. The result is that income differences appear narrower than they really are. So important is this effect, that in one data source there is now a significant correlation between low response rates in income surveys and the reported width of the income distribution. (High non-response rates mean that the tails of the income distribution are lost and narrower income distributions are reported.) Although there are ways of partially overcoming this problem, they do not give a better guide as to whether the figure we are interested in is 30 or 50 per cent of the population. These issues, which pose important problems for future research in this area, are discussed in more detail elsewhere (McIsaac and Wilkinson 1996).

There are numerous other problems of interpretation here. The income share received by the 30 or 50 per cent may be less important in its own right than as a proxy for the whole income distribution. But even if that were so, it would not tell us what was the best measure of overall income distribution – the Gini coefficient used in figure 5.6, the share of income going to the poorest so many per cent, or the proportion of the population living on less than some fraction such as half the average? Unfortunately the basic data are not strong enough to answer these questions. The US data probably have the best chance of resolving these issues. Not only are data available for fifty states, but they are less affected by low response rates.

The same is true in relation to questions about which equivalence scales should be used. Equivalence scales is the name given to the system used for adjusting aggregate household incomes to allow for the number of people living in each household. You could simply divide household income by the number of people in the household to get household income per capita. But as it is much cheaper for (say) four people to live together, sharing a washing machine, fridge, television, heating bills and the costs of services, it would seem appropriate to use an equivalence scale which took account of those kinds of economies. But clearly the economies of scale with things like heating costs are much greater than the economies of scale for the costs of food or clothing. Which is the more important for welfare is a matter of opinion: there is as yet no non-arbitrary way of choosing equivalence scales. My impression is that equivalence scales that emphasise the economies of scale gained by larger households, i.e. those that are furthest from per capita household income, tend to be most closely related to health. If the data were good enough, it might have been possible to use health to arbitrate between rival equivalence scales and show which gave the best guide to welfare. This would have made an important contribution to debates on the measurement of poverty and the setting of welfare benefits. Perhaps one day the quality of the data will have improved enough to enable that task to be tackled.

Returning to the issue of what proportion of the population's income share is most closely related to national mortality rates, we encounter another paradox. If it was the income share of a large proportion of the population – say 70 per cent – which mattered most, we would be confident that income distribution had effects on health spread widely across society. But if it turned out to be the income share received by the bottom 10 to 20 per cent which mattered most, we might still assume that the health effects were widespread on the grounds that changes in the mortality of the poorest 10 to 20 per cent alone could not have a large enough influence on national mortality rates. Their poverty would then seem to be affecting social life more widely.

The size of the differences in life expectancy between the more and less egalitarian countries provides another indication of the proportion of the population involved in this relationship. The differences are much too large to be accounted for by removing the mortality disadvantage of the proportion of the population classified as social class IV and V (semi and unskilled manual workers and their families). That would only produce about a quarter of the two years' difference in average life expectancy which separates the more from the less egalitarian countries in figure 5.3 or 5.6. This sounds like good evidence of a more widespread impact on mortality. But even here there is a serious problem. Measures of the size of mortality differences within a population are (as we saw in chapter 4) strongly influenced by the accuracy and appropriateness of the social classification which is used. We simply do not know how big mortality differences would be if an appropriate social classification were applied accurately to the whole population. Judging from the Whitehall study of civil servants, there seems no reason for thinking that differences would not be two or three times as large as the twofold differences shown in the official statistics for the economically active population. If that were so, then removing the mortality disadvantage of the bottom 30 per cent or so might make enough difference to average life expectancy.

The reader can now see the extent of the uncertainty. We know greater income equality increases average life expectancy, and we can be confident that this is at least partly, probably largely, because of an effect on health inequalities. The international relationship showing that health inequalities are wider where income differences are larger is evidence of that (Kunst and Mackenbach 1994; van Doorslaer *et al.* 1996). However, how low relative incomes have to be to affect health is not clear; nor is it clear to what extent health among the better-off may also benefit from what we might call the 'knock-on' effects of the reduction of relative deprivation elsewhere in that society.

So far we have looked almost exclusively at international data on income distribution and national mortality rates. Evidence of the way income inequality feeds into health inequalities and so into national mortality rates can be gleaned from evidence of change over time within Britain. However, looking at the relationship between annual changes in income distribution and annual changes in life expectancy in Britain is not the right approach. British income distribution data comes from the Family Expenditure Survey which, as well as having ordinary sampling error, has a non-response rate which is usually over 30 per cent. Because, in reality, income distribution changes very slowly, in most periods much of the annual change in reported income distribution will be derived from sampling error and variations in the scale of the bias introduced by non-response rates. On top of this there are some random fluctuations in annual life expectancy caused by such things as economic cycles, whether winter temperatures are higher or lower than usual, and passing epidemics of infectious diseases. The result is that correlating annual changes involves relating sampling error in income distribution figures to random fluctuations in life expectancy. Even if it were not for the noise in the system from these sources, allowances may need to be made for lag times before any relationships become apparent.

Although these problems mean that it is unlikely that any relationship can be found between annual changes in income distribution and mortality, they do not preclude the possibility that relationships can be found over longer periods, when the ratio of random noise to real changes recorded by the data is dramatically improved.

The best measures of social class differences in mortality over a long period are reworked figures based on the Registrar General's Decennial Supplements on Occupational Mortality available for 1921, 1931, 1951, 1961, 1971 and 1981 (Pamuk 1985). We saw in the last chapter how Pamuk made long-term measures of changing social class mortality differences. Her slope index of inequality measured differences across the whole population rather than just comparing extreme classes. She also allowed for the effects of the changing class classification of occupations and for the changing proportion of the population in each class. The results gave a surprisingly robust view of what has happened to social class differences in mortality. Essentially, mortality differences narrowed before the war to reach their narrowest in 1951 and have widened each decade since then, though the widening during the decade 1961–71 was very slight. This coincides fairly closely with what has happened to relative poverty (Wilkinson 1989). Although unemployment was high in 1931 it was fairly similar to the levels of unemployment in 1921 following demobilisation. However, the big difference between 1921 and 1931 reflects the dramatic growth of the welfare state with the introduction of unemployment insurance, sickness insurance and pensions. In relative terms the poor and the unemployed were much better off in 1931 than they were in 1921.

Because the social class classification of mortality is a classification only of the economically active population of working age (including the registered unemployed), the trends in poverty among the other groups of the population cannot be applied directly. Changes in poverty among the economically inactive are much less important than unemployment and the distribution of earnings.

By 1951 relative poverty and unemployment had been reduced to a fraction of prewar levels. The Second World War had seen the virtual elimination of unemployment and a dramatic narrowing in income differentials. The postwar Labour government had prevented the unemployment catastrophe which occurred immediately after the First World War, and the welfare state had been substantially expanded. The late 1940s and early 1950s probably saw Britain at its most egalitarian during peace time. A poverty survey conducted in the early 1950s found only about 8 per cent were in relative poverty. An estimate of a roughly comparable measure in the early 1990s would suggest that the proportion in relative poverty had at least tripled. Class differences in death rates also reached their narrowest on record in the 1951 figures. But from then on unemployment levels rose at a gradually accelerating rate, and health inequalities widened. The period 1951–61 saw a particularly dramatic widening of mortality differences as food rationing and a number of other postwar controls were removed. The National Food Survey shows that from the mid-1950s an increasing proportion of the population failed to reach recommended nutrient intake levels (Lambert 1964). Between 1953–4 and 1960 there was almost a 60 per cent increase in the proportion of the population living on less than 140 per cent of the old 'national assistance' standard. The deterioration was only slight during the 1960s but was again more marked over the period 1971–81. During the 1970s and 1980s unemployment grew particularly rapidly. Though dipping around 1975–6, relative poverty increase in the later 1970s and more rapidly in the 1980s – particularly in the later 1980s. There is then evidence of a rough fit between what happens to health inequalities and relative poverty among the economically active population during the years 1921–81 (Wilkinson 1989).

When the 1991 occupational mortality figures become available, they are likely to show the continued impact of increasing relative poverty. We can already see the effects of widening income differences on local disparities and on the rate of reduction in national mortality rates. Rather than the usual rather slow changes in income distribution, under Thatcher during the later 1980s income differences widened very rapidly. The trends are shown in figure 5.9. Both the Gini coefficient and the ratio of incomes of the bottom and top 20 per cent of the population shown in the figure record a slow widening of income differences until the mid-1980s and then, from about 1985 onwards, a more rapid widening. The rate at which inequality increased during this period is almost unprecedented. Among the OECD countries only New Zealand

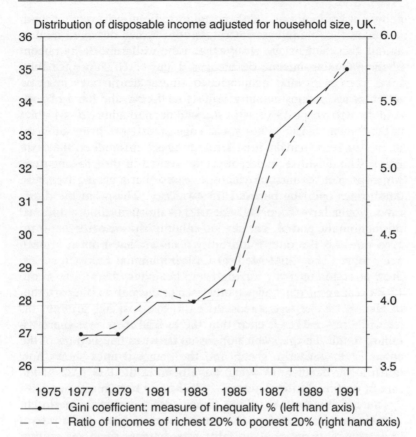

Figure 5.9 : Widening income differences: distribution of disposable income adjusted for household size, UK
Note: The Gini coefficient measures the degree of income inequality – not just between rich and poor, but across the whole population. The larger the coefficient, the greater the inequality. If everyone had the same income, the coefficient would be 0%. If all income went to one person and everyone else went without, the coefficient would be 100%.
Source: Central Statistical Office, *Economic Trends* 475: 129. 1993.
Acknowledgement to A.B. Atkinson

saw a faster widening of income differences (Hills 1994). Where economists used to discuss the mysterious long-term stability of income distribution, in the later 1980s the gap between rich and poor widened sufficiently rapidly to make it worth looking for an impact on annual mortality figures.

Most of the growth of income inequality took place among

people of working age and their children. Relative poverty among old people only increased very slightly during this period. It is among the younger age groups that we find the mortality impact of the widening income differences. Figure 5.10 shows for both sexes combined what happened to annual death rates in three different age groups: infant mortality in the bottom band of each column, children 1–19 years in the middle, and adults 20–44 years in the top band. The values in each age group have been set equal to 100 for 1985 to make it easier to compare them all on the same graph. The diagonal lines behind the columns are regression lines which project forward in each age group the declining trends in death rates over the period 1975–84. They show what the death rates would have been had the same rate of decline continued throughout the period. The shaded columns show clearly that from 1985 onwards the rate of mortality decline slowed down in each age group. (The Chief Medical Officer's annual report for 1990 drew attention to this worrying trend believing death rates in the 15–44 year age group had actually risen in this period (Department of Health 1991).) Age standardising in five-year age groups – as shown here – makes it clear that the overall trend was merely a failure to fall. The gap which opens up between the sections of the columns for each age group and the diagonal lines shows how much lower death rates would have been in the late 1980s if the rate of decline during the years 1975–84 had been maintained.

There is obviously a striking coincidence between the period of widening income differentials and the slowing down of the rate of improvement in national mortality rates in these three age groups. But is this mere coincidence? What other reasons are there for thinking that the two are causally related? Strong evidence that they are related comes from the results of three separate studies. They all compared changes in socioeconomic deprivation with changes in mortality rates for small areas in England or Scotland between the 1981 and 1991 censuses. They all found that socioeconomic differences between electoral wards had widened during the decade, and that this was matched by a widening of differentials in death rates. A study in Scotland found that death rates had increased during the decade among young men and women living in the more deprived post-code areas (McLoone and Boddy 1994). In the study (mentioned earlier) of 678 electoral wards in the Northern Region of England it was again found that death rates had increased among young adults living in the poorest wards (Phillimore *et al.* 1994).

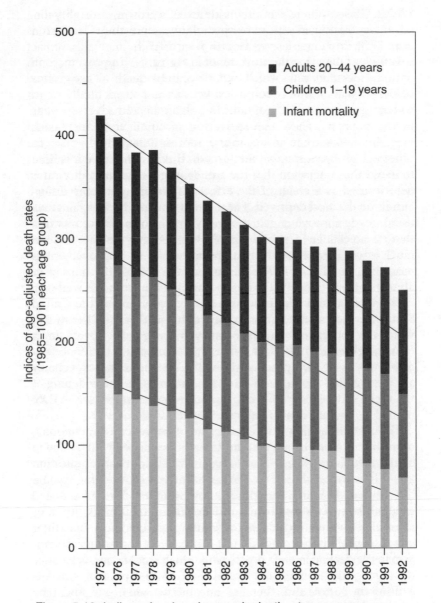

Figure 5.10: Indices showing changes in death rates among young adults, children and infants (M&F combined, England and Wales, 1975–92)
Source: Wilkinson 1994c

Within Glasgow there was also evidence of a growing mortality disadvantage associated with increasing relative deprivation (McCarron *et al*. 1994; Greater Glasgow Health Board 1993).

It is clear then that the slow down in the rate of improvement in national mortality rates which took place in Britain in all age groups below 45 years not only coincided with an unprecedentedly rapid widening of income differentials, but also reflected adverse trends in the poorest areas. As deprivation in these areas increased, mortality in some age groups in the poorest areas actually rose. In other age groups it simply failed to fall. But in either case it is hard to avoid the conclusion that the trends in national mortality rates deteriorated as a result of the effects of widening income differentials on the most deprived. These trends have to be set against the usual steady improvement in mortality which normally occurs when there is no change in income distribution. During the later 1980s a much larger proportion of the population saw no improvement in mortality, and the improvements among the better-off groups were almost entirely offset by the deterioration among the less well-off.

It is likely that similar processes affected mortality in the United States. As income differences widened during the 1980s the rate at which the population's life expectancy improved also slowed down (Kochanek *et al*. 1994). As figure 5.11 shows, the national slow down was associated particularly with a decline in life expectancy among the black population. Contributing most to the widening of the racial differences in life expectancy were heart disease, AIDS, homicide, and accidents (Kochanek *et al*. 1994).

To find that the slow down in the rate of improvement in national mortality rates in Britain and the US was associated with widening health inequalities suggests a partial answer to our earlier question about how widely shared are the health effects of widening income differences. Although we do not know whether more advantaged groups also saw a slow down in the decline in their mortality rates (American whites include poor whites), we do know that their increasing relative incomes do not cause a compensating acceleration in the decline in their death rates which would counterbalance the damage done among the less well-off. If relative income makes a difference to health, then, as an abstract idea, one might be surprised if increases in the relative incomes of those already at the top of the heap do not lead to more rapid improvements in their health. However, thinking about this in any practical context, there is no reason why the health of the rich should gain as a result of the

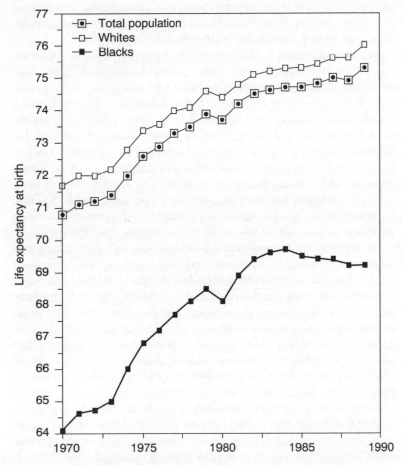

Figure 5.11: Trends in life expectancy among blacks and whites in the USA (M&F combined)
Source: Kochanek *et al*. 1994

increasing social tensions, despair and degeneration in the inner city areas. No one suggests that the health of the rich might in any way benefit from the fact that death rates in Harlem in New York are at most ages higher than in rural Bangladesh (McCord and Freeman 1990). The degeneration of such areas, usually associated with growing problems of crime, drugs and violence, is clearly a threat to the security and well-being of the population much more widely. One would therefore expect that while the main effect of income distribution on national mortality rates would come from its impact on the least well-off, there would also be some wider knock-on effects among the better-off.

In most research designs no distinction can be made between relative and absolute income. If one person's income is higher than another's, it is higher in both relative and absolute terms. Given that it is impossible to examine the effects of different living standards in socially isolated, Robinson Crusoe-like individuals, the only way we can distinguish the social effects of income differences from the asocial effects of material living standards *per se*, is to compare income differences within and between whole societies within which social comparisons are internal. This is what we did earlier when comparing life expectancy with GNPpc between countries and income distribution within them. It is after all societies, not individuals, which have income distributions.

Even though at the individual level it is impossible to distinguish relative from absolute income, it may be helpful to look briefly at the evidence from individual data that income – in whatever form – is indeed an important determinant of health. We have already seen two examples of data which show strong cross-sectional associations. One, shown in figure 5.1, p. 73, was of mortality using data from the MRFIT study (Davey Smith *et al.* 1996). The other was the association between income and self-reported illness reported in nine different countries by van Doorslaer *et al.* (1996) (see p. 88). But uncontrolled associations tell us little about causality. The Alameda County Study which followed up a population in California, found that income was closely related to health even after controlling for seven other health-related factors (Slater *et al.* 1985). However, it is always possible to argue that the rich differ from the poor in ways that are too subtle to be effectively measured and controlled. Even if a group of people are the same with respect – for instance – to education, health-related behaviour and social class, it could still be imagined that the richer ones would be healthier because they have more initiative or whatever, which has not been measured. The same can be said even if you study individuals over time as they become richer or poorer: there may still be unrecognised differences between those who became richer or poorer.

One piece of research which attempted to get round some of these problems did so by studying the effects of income changes for which people were not, in some sense, self-selected. It looked to see if there was a relationship between changes in the incomes and death rates of people between 1971 and 1981 in some sixty-four different occupational groups which could be identified at each end of the period (Wilkinson 1990). The question was whether the changing positions of occupations in the occupational mortality 'league table' were related to changes in their position in the occupational earnings league. In general, changing earnings differentials between occupational groups will be determined by impersonal economic forces, changing technology, market position and international competition, rather than by the personal characteristics of the individuals in those occupations. The only methodological problem with this research design was that if occupations moved significantly up or down the earnings league, it might cause some selective recruitment or loss of people from those occupations. Whether, as an occupation sinks, it is the least healthy who are made redundant first, or the healthy who leave early to take better jobs, is not clear. But it was possible to control for changes in the size of occupations which would take account of either selective process – whatever their effects. One other refinement was to restrict comparisons to the same cohort in each occupation as they aged during the decade. This meant comparing – for example – people in their thirties or forties in each occupation in 1971 with those who were in their forties or fifties in 1981. It is likely that this helped to ensure that a large proportion of the same individuals were included in the comparison at each point in time: even if someone changed employers several times, most teachers would remain teachers and most train drivers would remain train drivers. The research results showed clearly that changes in an occupation's position in the mortality league was significantly related to changes in the proportion of people in that occupation who were unemployed or had low earnings. Increases in the proportion unemployed and in the proportion with low earnings were independently related to a deterioration in the position of an occupation in the mortality league.

There has been one genuinely randomised control trial of the effects of income change. It was set up to examine the economic and social effects of a proposed system of negative income tax in Gary, Indiana (Kehrer and Wolin 1979). Unfortunately the only health outcomes which were measured were pregnancy and childbirth. The study focused exclusively on a low-income population who were randomised between continuing in the ordinary welfare system or receiving negative income tax. The group receiving negative income tax ended up with incomes averaging about 50 per cent more than families in the control group. The study found that, in each of four groups of women at high risk of having low-birthweight babies, the women receiving negative income tax had significantly heavier babies.

It is usually assumed that the connection between this kind of evidence, suggesting that income is causally related to health, and a relationship between average health and income distribution, depends on showing that changes in income have a bigger effect on the health of the poor than they do on the health of the rich. I initially thought that it was only worth looking for a relationship between income distribution and national mortality rates if this was so. The question seemed to be whether the income–mortality relationship was curved in such a way that taking £100 from the rich and adding it to the incomes of the poor would increase the health of the poor by more than it decreased the health of the rich.

The evidence from the analysis of changes in occupational incomes and mortality rates (discussed above) had suggested that mortality rates were only affected by changes in the proportion of people in each occupation on low incomes. As well as the evidence from the analysis of changes over the decade 1971–81, the cross-sectional relationship between occupational incomes and mortality was also curved so as to suggest that mortality among those less well-off was more responsive to changes in income than it was among the better-off. Finally, among 9,000 people covered in the Health and Lifestyles Survey, three measures of self-reported illness showed not simply a curved relationship with income but a relationship which suggested that, after falling rates of illness as you moved up the income scale from the poor, there was a tendency for illness rates actually to increase again as you moved from the middle income range to the rich – a reverse 'J' shaped curve suggesting that if the rich got richer they would get iller (Blaxter 1990). There had been a similar suggestion from the USA of poorer health illness among the richest (Grossman 1972). This held out the remarkable – if implausible – prospect that income transfers from the rich to the poor might improve the health of both simultaneously. However, Mildred Blaxter has since pointed out that the evidence of rising illness rates among the rich is based on very small numbers, mainly from a few wealthy young men and some rich widows, and so may not be a reliable guide to the relationship among the rich more generally (personal communication).

There is also some evidence suggesting not only that health shows no sign of deterioration at high income levels, but that the relationship is not even curved. The US data from the MRFIT study shown in figure 5.1 indicate an uncompromisingly linear relationship. (It should however be borne in mind that the income data in this study is the average income in the zip code area in which each person lives rather than their own individual income.) If the causal relationship were linear, a $1,000 reduction in the incomes of the rich would harm their health by just as much as a $1,000 increase would improve the health of the poor. There would be no net benefit from income redistribution. There have since been several other studies of the shape of the relationship between income and health. Backlund et al. reported a curved relationship with mortality in the USA (Backlund et al. 1996).

In case this equivocal picture reflected the influence of various technical problems, it seemed worth looking at the issue exclusively among a group of people among whom the technical problems would be minimised. First, by confining attention to the retired population it would reduce the element of reverse causality by which working people who become sick may suffer a drop in earnings. In general the retired population have pensions fixed independently of their health. Using data kindly supplied by Sara Arber from the *General Household Survey*, we excluded incomes from invalidity benefit and attendance allowances which serve to increase the incomes of the sick elderly. Second, because of the problems discussed earlier of the arbitrary choice of equivalence scales to use when adjusting household income to take account of the number of people in each household, it seemed best to confine the analysis to the large number of households containing just one or two old people, and to analyse these two groups separately. But, as luck would have it, even on this squeaky-clean basis, the self-reported morbidity measures taken from the *General Household Survey* in Britain gave no clear-cut verdict. An example of the results is shown in figure 5.12. The relationship is neither coherently linear nor non-linear. However, given that the data for the lowest income group in any income survey tend to be unreliable because a number of fairly well-off people living on capital or savings and spending more than the average tend to say they have

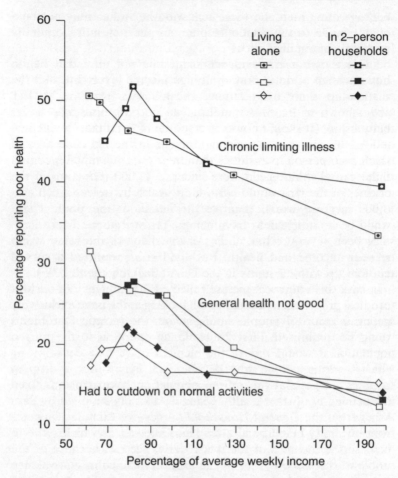

Figure 5.12: Three measures of self-reported health in relation to income among men and women (combined) 65 years and over living alone or in two-person households
Source: Data from *General Household Survey* provided by Sara Arber

no income or sometimes even negative incomes, the relationship might tend towards a curve. If it were possible to take these people with low declared incomes and yet high living standards out of the lowest income group, the illness rate among the remaining genuinely poor might be high enough to give a more convincing picture of a curved relationship.

Having run their course, the arguments in these areas have now been almost turned on their heads. Rather than the plausibility of a relationship between income distribution and population mortality being dependent on establishing that the relationship between individual income and health is curved, the income distribution relationship is now firmly established – regardless of the shape of the individual relationship. Similarly, we can be considerably more confident that there is some kind of causal relationship between income equity and average mortality than we can that individual incomes are a real determinant of health. Although the latter seems highly plausible and there is some evidence to suggest that it is true, there is very little evidence which is proof against the criticism that it merely shows the effects of self-selection. On the other hand, because the income distribution relationship deals with whole populations, it is not vulnerable to selective mechanisms.

Now that the shape of the income–health relationship has refused to reveal itself unequivocally, it has became clear that its curvature is not a necessary precondition for the influence of income distribution on health. It was George Davey Smith (who produced the data for the linear relationship in figure 5.1) who first persuaded me – over coffee outside Glasgow Central Station – to think about how linearity could be consistent with an effect of income distribution.

Underlying the idea that the relationship must be curved is the economist's notion of the declining marginal utility of increases in income. Basically this is simply the idea that once you have lots of something – say food – then more is less useful to you than it would be to someone with less. Poorer people are more likely to have unmet needs that affect their health than are the rich. But underlying this line of reasoning is still the notion that it is absolute levels of consumption that matter: that it is the utility of the goods (or services) themselves which count, and this utility which varies between rich and poor. However, if we think in wholly relative terms, things work rather differently. What matters is not the nature of the goods themselves as much as the social connotations of different income and consumption levels. Measures of relative income would always have to be based on a reference point in each society. That reference point is commonly taken as the average income – hence relative poverty is usually defined in terms of the proportion of the population living on less than 50 per cent of the average income. But, to clarify the argument about curvature, let us take a different reference point. Imagine measuring all social position and hierarchy in relation to the top 10 per cent, and taking income differences as a measure of everyone else's distance below that top 10 per cent. Let us also assume that the further people's incomes are below the norms of the top 10 per cent, the more their health suffers. It would then be possible to have an entirely linear relationship between income and health in each society and yet find that overall health improved as income differences narrowed. Narrower income differences would reduce the extent of the health-damaging social disadvantage in relation to the top 10 per cent.

As a model this has some credibility. In addition to the positive correlations between life expectancy and the income shares of the lower deciles, there is always a negative correlation with the share of the top 10 per cent (the bigger the share of society's income going to the top 10 per cent, the lower is average life expectancy). The model's use of a relative income concept which, whatever the incomes of the top 10 per cent, never allows them to do better than the best (i.e. the reference point at which incomes equal 1) would also explain why the health effects of worsening relative incomes lower down the scale are not offset by any benefits of increasing advantage higher up the scale. It looks therefore as if by taking income in wholly relative terms, and assuming that what damages health is something to do with socioeconomic disadvantage itself, that the effect of income distribution on average health could be consistent even with a linear relationship between income and health within a society. If this is the case, perhaps the most appropriate measure of income distribution to use in relation to health would be analogous to the mechanics of leverage, summing the moments of force round a fulcrum or reference point. Taking a reference point such as the incomes of the top 10 per cent, the total force of relative deprivation in a society would be measured by summing the proportionate income distances of everyone else below the reference group. The finding that the so-called 'Robin Hood' index of inequality (which measures the maximum distance between the Lorenz curve and the line of income equality) is more closely related than the Gini coefficient to mortality among the fifty states of the USA suggests that this might be the way to proceed (Kennedy *et al.* 1996).

The evidence allows us to go no further. Whether the relationship between income and health is linear or curved remains unknown: there is evidence on both sides. That it is not indisputably curved is perhaps an indication that it is not sufficiently curved for the curvature to be the main source of the life expectancy–income distribution relationship. However, it is only when using concepts appropriate to the influence of absolute income levels on health that a curvilinear relationship is implied by the effect of income distribution. If we think instead of the impact of relative income on health, and define relative income levels in genuinely relative terms, then even a linear relationship between income and health within countries would be consistent with the effects of income distribution on national mortality rates. The debate then becomes irrelevant.

Another point at which the concepts of relative and absolute income need to be more clearly distinguished is in interpreting the size of the differences in income share associated with several years' difference in average national life expectancy. Typically a difference of only about 7 per cent in the share of income going to the bottom 50 per cent of the population is associated with something like a two year increase in life expectancy (Wilkinson 1994b). This looks too small a change in income to provide a plausible explanation of the difference in life expectancy. The figures are set out in table 5.1. The top row shows the shares of total income which might be received by the bottom and top 50 per cent of the population in some of the less egalitarian of the developed societies: 27 and 73 per cent respectively. (Together these must of course add up to 100 per cent of the society's personal disposable income.) The second row shows the shares which might typically be found in more egalitarian societies: 7 per cent has been added to the share of the bottom half, bringing it up to 34 per cent. As a consequence, the share of the top half has declined from 73 to 66 per cent. However, although the difference is only 7 per cent, if one calculates the ratio of incomes in the bottom half relative to the top half (last column of table 5.1) it turns out that the relative income of the bottom half has increased from 37 per cent to 52 per cent of what the top half get. This represents more than a 40 per cent increase in their relative incomes. Although a calculation which turns a 7 per cent increase into a 40 per cent increase might seem to involve some sleight-of-hand, it is clear that the first figure is the change in the absolute income levels, whereas the second is a calculation based consistently on the logic of relative income.

Having surveyed a number of issues to do with the statistical evidence on the relationship between income and health, we can begin to see a fairly coherent picture. The main features are as

Table 5.1: The effect of different distributions of income on the relative income of the poorest half of the population

	Bottom 50% of pop.	Top 50% of pop.	Ratio of bottom to top
% shares of total income (A)	27	73	0.37 : 1
% shares of total income (B)	34	66	0.52 : 1
Percentage increase (A to B) of *relative income* of bottom 50%:-			**40.5**

Note: The table shows how a 7 per cent increase (from 27% to 34%) in the share of income received by the poorest 50 per cent of the population results in a 40 per cent increase in their relative income.

follows. First, there is some quite good evidence – and it is highly plausible – that health is responsive to changes in income. Second, there are a number of powerful reasons for thinking that relative income is more important than absolute income in the rich developed countries. These include the evidence that the epidemiological transition marks the achievement of living standards among the bulk of the population adequate to ensure that basic needs are no longer the primary constraint on the population's health. It also includes the apparent paradox of the close relationship between income and health within developed countries and the lack of any such relationship between developed countries. Providing strong confirmation of the relative income interpretation of this paradox is the relationship between income inequality and average life expectancy which has been shown to exist in both rich and poor countries. This has now been demonstrated cross-sectionally and on data dealing with changes over time, and the relationship cannot be plausibly attributed to some intervening variable. There is also evidence that the scale of income differences in developed countries is related to the scale of health inequalities within them. This appears to be true in cross-country comparisons as well as within countries over time. The implication is that income inequalities influence national mortality rates primarily by determining the strength of the impact of relative deprivation on health. Whether the health of the better-off also improves as income differences narrow is not clear, but it is clear that changes in income differences do not lead to changes in the health of the rich which substantially offset the changes in the health of the poor. Hence narrowing health inequalities give rise to faster improvements in national mortality rates. The fact that health inequalities have not shown any general tendency to narrow in developed countries during the course of economic development implies that they are not a reflection of absolute poverty.

The powerful effects of relative income and their inherently social nature present a formidable challenge to conventional economics which has based itself largely on maximising the asocial pleasures of material consumption. The extent to which social needs are primary and must be taken into account by the system through which society satisfies its material needs has not been adequately addressed by economic science. Although economics is far from exclusively asocial, the weight of the application of rational choice theory has grossly underestimated human social needs and the fact that their satisfaction should often take precedence, particularly in affluent societies, over the demands to maximise individual consumption. There is a missing social economy of well-being.

Part III

Social cohesion and social conflict

Chapter 6

A small town in the USA, wartime Britain, Eastern Europe and Japan

What seems to be one of the most important distinctions between the way relative and absolute income impact on health is that absolute income will affect health through the direct physiological effects of material circumstances, whereas relative income involves inherently social elements in the causal processes. Absolute income may affect health through exposure to toxic materials, through a poor diet, damp housing and inadequate heating. The powerful influence which relative income seems to have suggests that it is not so much a matter of what your circumstances are in themselves, but of their standing in relation to others: of where they place you in the overall scale of things, and of the impact which this has on your psychological, emotional and social life. We shall get on to those issues in chapters 8, 9 and 10. But rather than going from the concept of income distribution (in the last chapter) directly to the pathways through which individual relative income may determine individual health, it would be useful to look briefly at the way wider social structures have been associated with narrower income differences and better health. We shall discuss five examples.

BRITAIN IN WARTIME

Much the most rapid improvements in life expectancy in Britain during the twentieth century came during the two world wars (Winter 1988). The increase in civilian life expectancy during each decade of the century is shown in table 6.1. In the decades which include the two world wars, life expectancy increased by between six and seven years for both men and women. This is well over twice as fast as the average rate of improvement during the rest of the century.

Table 6.1: Increases in life expectancy in England and Wales each decade 1901–91 (Additional years' life expectancy at birth)

	1901/11	1911/21	1921/31	1931/40	1940/51	1951/60	1961/71	1971/81	1981/91
Men	4.1	6.6	2.3	1.2	6.5	2.4	0.9	2.0	2.4
Women	4.0	6.5	2.4	1.5	7.0	3.2	1.2	1.8	2.0

Sources: S.H. Preston, N. Keyfitz and R. Schoen *Causes of Death. Life tables for national populations*. Academic Press, N.Y. 1972; OPCS, *Population Trends*, HMSO, London. 1995.

Both wars were periods which saw a massive diversion of production from civilian consumption to production for the war effort. Living standards ceased to rise and, especially as a result of bombing during the Second World War, housing standards deteriorated. Medical services were also diverted from civilian use on a vast scale to meet the needs of wounded soldiers. Although food rationing improved the quality of the nation's diet during the Second World War and is often given the credit for the health improvements, such an explanation ignores the fact that it does not apply to the First World War. Both wars however saw a return to full employment and a dramatic narrowing of income differences. Winter describes the attempt to ensure basic minimum standards for all, which he says led to a levelling up of health standards, with the most rapid improvements coming in the poorest areas (Winter 1985, 1988). Not only did unemployment virtually disappear, but differences in earnings amongst those in employment narrowed very substantially.

> What changed [during the First World War] was both an enhancement of the market position of most grades of manual labour as well as a strengthening of the legal and moral entitlement of workers to exchange their labour for a living wage.
>
> (Winter 1985, p. 244)

Winter says 'primary poverty among the urban and rural poor was an unexpected casualty of the war' (p. 245). He also remarks on the consequential 'drop in indictments and convictions for theft and other offences as well as a decline in vagrancy and recourse to the Poor Law relief' (p. 245).

While the narrowing of income differences during the Second World War was partly a labour market response to the shortage of labour, it was also pursued as a deliberate policy. As Titmuss said in his essay 'War and Social Policy': 'If the cooperation of the masses was thought to be essential [to the war effort], then inequalities had to be reduced and the pyramid of social stratification had to be flattened' (Titmuss 1958, p. 86). The Beveridge Report, which was commissioned in June 1941 and reported less than 18 months later in November 1942, was part of this attempt. Its plans for a massive expansion of the welfare state were part of the morale-boosting aim of creating a 'nation fit for heroes'. Given the heavy burden which the war imposed on government expenditure, there could be no other reason to choose 1941 as the moment to consider plans for the dramatic expansion of welfare expenditure.

The protection of the population from the rigours of scarcity mediated by the market involved not only the rationing of food and many other goods including clothes, furniture, petrol and coal, but also a system of price controls and subsidies.

As well as the disappearance of unemployment during the Second World War, there was also a dramatic reduction of income differentials. Calculations suggest that while real post-tax incomes increased by more than 9 per cent among those identified by Seers as working class, they fell by more than 7 per cent among the middle class (Milward 1984 p. 41). Comparisons of the Seebohm Rowntree surveys of poverty in York in 1936 with Rowntree and Laver in 1950 suggest that rates of relative poverty were halved between those dates (Townsend 1979).

Life during the war is always described in terms of the sense of camaraderie, of people pulling together and a sense of social cohesion. This sense of unity had three sources: first, there was the psychological sense of unity in the face of a common enemy. Second were the market conditions which reduced unemployment, income differences, and the social divisions which go with them. Third was a deliberate policy designed to foster a sense of social unity and co-operation in the war effort. It is impossible to tell how much each of these different components contributed. Indeed, what is interesting is the snowballing effect as each strengthened the others. The desire to share the costs of war fairly fitted well with the need to raise revenue by taxing those who could afford to pay: the inevitable result was a narrowing of post-tax income differentials. The reduction of unemployment removed a source of social division and bitterness at the same time as giving people a role in a common task. Although such exogenous decreases in the economic causes of social division may often lead to a greater sense of social cohesion, during the war there were also exogenous social and political factors adding to the sense of unity which may then have fed back into a greater willingness to reduce the economic divisions.

In the war at least some of the usual sequence of causation, running from economic to social divisions, may have been reversed. By the end of the war there was certainly a desire to create a society which took better care of its members. As well as the deliberate creation of policy, this was also fed by the actual experience of smaller distinctions and a common purpose among the population. This no doubt contributed to the victory of the Labour Party in the 1945 general election. In a similar vein, it is interesting to speculate whether the widening income differences and social divisions under Thatcher, the increasing sense of insecurity as public services were weakened, actually encouraged a retreat into individualism and conservatism which led to the succession of Conservative election victories in the 1980s and early 1990s.

The example of wartime Britain illustrates the possibility that income distribution may serve as a proxy for a number of important aspects of society related to social cohesion. While income distribution is too closely related to health to believe that it is merely a distant marker for other 'real' determinants of health, it is important to see income differentials as enmeshed in wider patterns of ideology and social and economic relations which both determine it and are determined by it. The deterioration of absolute material standards for much of the population also pinpoints the need to see the dramatic improvement in civilian death rates as intimately related to greater equity.

ROSETO, PENNSYLVANIA

As a small town of some 1,600 people, Roseto, in eastern Pennsylvania, attracted attention for its low death rates – particularly from heart attacks (Bruhn and Wolf 1979). Research has shown that death rates were substantially lower than neighbouring towns from as early as the mid-1930s. The fact that death rates from heart disease were initially over 40 per cent lower in Roseto was not explained by the usual risk factors such as diet, smoking and exercise (Wolf and Bruhn 1993).

The population was largely made up of Italian-Americans descended from migrants who arrived during a large-scale emigration in the 1880s from the Italian town of Roseto on the

Eastern side of southern Italy. After failing to explain the health differences in terms of known risk factors, researchers' attention was caught by how much more closely knit was the community in Roseto, Pennsylvania, than that in neighbouring towns. It was said to be characterised by 'close family ties and cohesive community relationships' (Egolf *et al.* 1992, p. 1089). There are a number of indications that the increased social cohesion of Roseto was accompanied by an egalitarian ethos. Bruhn and Wolf remarked:

> The local priest emphasised that when the preoccupation with earning money exceeded the unmarked boundary it became the basis for social rejection, irrespective of the standing of the person . . . During the first five years of our study [i.e. from 1961] it was difficult to distinguish, on the basis of dress or behaviour, the wealthy from the impecunious in Roseto. Living arrangements – houses and cars – were simple and strikingly similar. Despite the affluence of many, there was no atmosphere of 'keeping up with the Joneses'.
>
> (Bruhn and Wolf 1979, pp. 80, 81–2)

On the same theme, Bruhn and Wolf wrote:

> From the beginning the sense of common purpose and the camaraderie among the Italians precluded ostentation or embarrassment to the less affluent, and the concern for neighbors ensured that no one was ever abandoned. This pattern of remarkable social cohesion, in which the family, as the hub and bulwark of life, provided a kind of security and insurance against any catastrophe, was associated with the striking absence of myocardial infarction and sudden death.
>
> (ibid., p. 136)

The same point is emphasised repeatedly: 'Throughout the years of study of this community the indications were that the strength of unconditional interpersonal support and family and community cohesiveness had served to counteract the effects of life stress and thereby were a protection against fatal myocardial infarction' (ibid., p. 118).

As the community ties began to loosen in the 1960s, and young people began to move away, the researchers correctly predicted that Roseto would lose its health advantage. Commenting on the process of change they wrote:

The gradual abandonment of the old ways in Roseto . . . was evident in the emerging preoccupation with materialistic values that accompanied increased education and growing affluence. During the decade from 1966–75 (when the health advantage disappeared) many Cadillacs and other expensive cars appeared on Roseto streets. . . . Their attraction to status symbols – expensive clothes, large automobiles, and elaborate new homes furnished on the advice of interior decorators – reflected the beginning [of the] breakdown of former egalitarian standards among Rosetans.

(ibid., pp. 111, 115–16)

The community had had a considerable health advantage which seemed explicable only in terms of its social characteristics. It was predicted that as it lost these characteristics it would lose its health advantage, and this seems to have been what happened. The researchers concluded:

The data obtained over a span of twenty years in the Italian-American community of Roseto, when compared with those of neighboring communities, strongly suggests that the cultural characteristics – the qualities of a social organization – affect in some way individual susceptibility to myocardial infarction and sudden death. The implication is that an emotionally supportive social environment is protective and that, by contrast, the absence of family and community support and the lack of a well-defined role in society are risk factors.

(ibid., p. 134)

Although the initial settlement by poor immigrants meant that there was some material basis to Roseto's social cohesion right from the beginning, it is clear that this is an example where an egalitarian ethos was maintained socially – at least for a while. However, one has the impression that the material and social can never drift too far apart. To maintain social cohesion involved minimising signs of material differences 'in dress, speech or manner' (p. 110). When the breakdown came, social cohesion gave way to ostentatious display.

THE REGIONS OF ITALY

A third example of the way social systems can work, which may throw light on the relationship between income distribution and health, comes by chance from a comparative study of the regions of Italy itself.

In 1970 new regional governments were set up in the twenty regions of Italy. Over the following two decades Putnam, Leonardi and Nanetti studied how effectively they worked and tried to explain the differences they found. The outline that follows is taken almost wholly from their book *Making democracy work: civic traditions in modern Italy*.

Putnam's measure of how well the new regional governments performed was an index based upon a dozen different factors including the governments' effectiveness in providing a wide range of services (housing, day care, family health clinics, etc.), their responsiveness to postal and telephone enquiries, the quality of their legislative record, and their promptness in approving annual budgets. The results showed large differences in governmental effectiveness with a general tendency for performance to be better in the more northerly regions than in the southern ones. As all the regional governments were funded at the same level of income per head of population, Putnam sought to explain the differences in terms of the characteristics of the regions themselves.

His first observation was that although the regions could be divided into a richer group and a poorer group and performance was better in the former than the latter, *within* either group there was no connection between income levels and performance. The explanation eventually developed from the statistical analysis was that local government functioned best in regions in which the 'civic community' was strong. The concept of civic community was the converse of 'self-interested (or sometimes 'a-moral') familism', terms which Putnam took from Banfield (1958). He measured regions on a scale which, at one extreme, had communities in which there was little or no involvement in public affairs unless in pursuit of the direct self-interest of oneself or one's family. In these areas where civic community was weakest, social relations were predominantly hierarchical and based on patronage. Public projects which would have been widely beneficial were often not undertaken because of a lack of a sense of civic responsibility and a grudging suspicion of the motives of anyone who did get involved.

At the other end of Putnam's scale were areas with well-developed civic communities, with a high level of awareness of and involvement in public affairs, in which the prevailing ethos was much more egalitarian and democratic. To measure people's involvement in public life, Putnam developed an index of the strength of civic community based on things like the percentage of the population voting in referenda, newspaper readership, and the number of associations for voluntary, cultural and sporting activities per head of population. The correlation between this index and his measure of government performance was 0.92, suggesting that well over three-quarters of the differences in performance could be accounted for by differences in the strength of the community.

After looking at the correlations among a range of other social attributes, Putnam summarised the contrast between regions with high and low levels of civic community:

> Some regions of Italy have many choral societies and soccer teams and bird-watching clubs and Rotary clubs. Most citizens in these regions read eagerly about community affairs in the daily press. They are engaged by public issues. . . . Inhabitants trust one another to act fairly and to obey the law. Leaders in these regions are relatively honest. They believe in popular government, and they are predisposed to compromise with their political adversaries. Both citizens and leaders here find equality congenial. Social and political networks are organised horizontally, not hierarchically. The community values solidarity, civic engagement, co-operation, and honesty. Government works. Small wonder that people in these regions are content!
>
> At the other pole are the 'uncivic' regions, aptly characterised by the French term *incivisme*. Public life in these regions is organised hierarchically, rather than horizontally. The very concept of 'citizen' here is stunted. From the point of view of the individual inhabitant, public affairs is the business of somebody else – *i notabili*, 'the bosses', 'the politicians' – but not me. Few people aspire to partake in deliberations about the common-weal, and few such opportunities present themselves. Political participation is triggered by personal dependency and private greed, not by collective purpose. Engagement in social and cultural associations is meagre. Private piety stands in for public purpose. Corruption is widely regarded as the norm, even by politicians themselves, and they are cynical about democratic principles. 'Compromise' has only negative overtones. Laws (almost everyone agrees) are made to be broken, but fearing

others' lawlessness, people demand sterner discipline. Trapped in these interlocking vicious circles, nearly everyone feels powerless, exploited and unhappy. All things considered, it is hardly surprising that representative government here is less effective than in more civic communities.

(Putnam *et al.* 1993, p. 115)

Although the characteristics of civic communities will vary from one society to another, Putnam's evidence shows that the strength of community life is an important variable. While he was interested in neither health nor income distribution, his work is relevant to them because civic community is in fact related to both. He mentions in a footnote that the correlation between his index of civic community and a narrower income distribution is 0.81 (p<0.001) – showing that there is a close and statistically significant relationship between them. He also mentions that there is correlation between stronger civic community and lower infant mortality rates. In addition, I have found a statistically significant relationship between his measures of civic community and female but not male life expectancy. Why male and female life expectancy should have different patterns of variation across the Italian regions is not clear, but it may represent the influence of other factors on male cardiovascular diseases.

This example once again shows that income distribution may be related to much more than the different amounts of money in people's pockets. As with the examples of state-planned economies (see below) and Britain during the wars, the Italian regions show that much wider issues to do with the social fabric of society are at stake. It is interesting to note that despite coming from an area characterised by its 'a-moral familism', the Italian migrants who set up the new Roseto ended up establishing such a closely knit community.

EASTERN EUROPE DURING THE 1970s AND 1980s

(Parts of this section are reproduced from Wilkinson 1996.)

Another arena which illustrates some rather different possibilities of these structural relations is provided by the former centrally planned, or state capitalist, countries of Eastern Europe and the

Third World. Since the early 1970s – long before the 1989 uprisings – life expectancy in Eastern Europe and the Soviet Union has failed to improve and has trailed further and further behind standards in Western Europe. However, until the early 1970s health in these countries was broadly comparable with health in Western Europe. Countries such as East Germany, Bulgaria and Romania did particularly well, indeed, life expectancy was higher in East than in West Germany. High standards of health had been achieved in Eastern Europe despite much lower living standards usually associated with less good health.

There can be little doubt that the standards of health in Eastern Europe up to the early 1970s provide an illustration of the broader pattern according to which more egalitarian countries, at all levels of development, had much better health than other countries at similar levels of GNPpc. Amartya Sen, writing in 1981, looked at improvements in life expectancy among 100 developed and less developed countries between 1960 and 1977 (Sen 1981). Because it is probably easier to add additional years of life expectancy in countries where it is initially low than it is in countries where it is already high, Sen measured progress by using the percentage decrease in the amount by which life expectancy fell short of 80 years. Between 1960 and 1977 he found that nine out of the ten communist countries in his list of 100 nations came within the top quarter for the percentage reduction they achieved in their life expectancy shortfall. The nine were Albania, Bulgaria, Romania and Yugoslavia from Eastern Europe, as well as Vietnam, China, N. Korea, Mongolia and Cuba. Only Hungary (perhaps significantly with its uprising in 1956 and subsequent purges) failed to make such rapid progress. As Sen remarks, 'One thought that is bound to occur (to anyone looking at his table of results) is that communism is good for poverty removal).'

Among the other countries which came within the top 25 per cent were El Salvador, Malaysia, Taiwan, Costa Rica, Hong Kong and Greece. The obvious link between some of these and the communist countries is their success in reducing relative poverty. Some achieved this mainly by narrowing income differences and others by effectively sharing the benefits of rapid economic growth throughout society.

Among less developed countries, and indeed in Central and Eastern Europe until the early 1970s, it appears that communism was good for health. Nor were the achievements of Eastern

Europe simply a matter of ensuring high levels of child immunisation and baby care. Even at the age of 15, life expectancy in
Eastern European countries was high compared with countries
with equally low levels of GNP per capita. Assuming for the
moment that 'communism' used to appear good for health through
some process related to narrower income differences and lower
levels of relative poverty, the question which then arises is what
went wrong? Why did improvements in life expectancy in Eastern
Europe cease in the early 1970s?

There are several important features of the failure of health
standards to rise any further. First the pattern is coterminous with
the political boundary between Eastern and Western Europe. In
terms of the death rates of men of working age, although there was
a considerable overlap between Eastern and Western Europe in
1970, by 1990 not one Eastern European country had death rates
lower than a single Western European country (Watson 1995). As
if to reflect its halfway political position, death rates in Yugoslavia
put it exactly in the middle between the two bloc. While Western
European countries continued to enjoy substantial improvements
in life expectancy, gains were small or non-existent in almost every
country in the former Soviet sphere of influence. Interestingly,
Albania – which was allied with China rather than the Soviet Union
– was the only country in Eastern Europe where life expectancy
continued to make significant improvements. This shows how
closely health is related to the political environment. Indeed,
looking at the trends in life expectancy in Eastern Europe, one has
a strong impression that if we knew why health failed to improve
after the early 1970s, we would also know the underlying causes
of the uprisings of 1989. Something went wrong in those societies
in the early 1970s and health is probably the clearest indicator
of it.

Several causes can be excluded. In his report for the World Bank,
Hertzman shows that Eastern Europe's poor health performance
cannot be explained in terms of any deterioration in standards of
medical care or of factors such as air pollution (Hertzman 1995).
Although air pollution is severe in some industrial areas, not enough
of the population is exposed for it to have significant effects on
national mortality rates. An interesting indication of the sociological nature of the cause we are seeking is Watson's observation
of the remarkable difference in mortality trends among single and
married people (Watson 1995). She showed that while there were

only small changes in death rates among married men and women during the years 1970–88 in Poland, there were very substantial increases among divorced men and women. A similar pattern has also been found in Hungary. During the 1970s and 1980s the increases in Hungarian premature mortality were greatest among men who were divorced, but were also marked among those who were widowed or had never married. Married men were relatively protected. Among women the greatest increases in death rates were among widows (Hajdu et al. 1995).

The effect on life expectancy of continued improvements in infant mortality rates was offset by increases in adult mortality rates, particularly among men. Although mortality rates did not rise significantly among married people, we might have expected them to fall among all sections of the population. The importance of the single–married dichotomy is not that the married were untouched by the causes we are looking for, merely that they had a differential effect according to marital status. This not only rules out general environmental influences such as air pollution, to which the whole population would be exposed, but also many society-wide economic influences, such as changes in the standard of living. (In fact, economic growth continued in the majority of Eastern European countries during most of the 1970s and 1980s.)

Probably one of the clearest descriptions of what went wrong in these societies was given by Gorbachev in his speech to the Central Committee of the Soviet Communist Party on 27 January 1987. In an extraordinary appeal for the Party to renew its social and moral commitment, he spoke of the 'loss of momentum', 'stagnation', and of 'unresolved problems piling up', which 'seriously affected the economy and the social and spiritual spheres'. He blamed the Party saying:

> vigorous debates and creative ideas [had] disappeared . . . while authoritarian evaluations and opinions became unquestionable truths . . . The social goals of the economy in the past few five-year plan periods were diluted and there emerged a deafness to the social issues . . . Elements of social corrosion which emerged in the past few years had a negative effect on society's morale, and somehow, unnoticed, eroded the lofty moral values which have always been characteristic of our people . . . [I]interest in the affairs of society slackened, manifestations of callousness and scepticism appeared . . .

The stratum of people, some of them young people, whose ultimate goal in life was material well-being and gain by any means, grew wider. Their cynical stand was acquiring more and more aggressive forms, poisoning the mentality of those around them, and triggering a wave of consumerism. The spread of alcohol and drug abuse, and a rise in crime, became indicators of the decline of social mores.

Disregard for laws, distortion of reports, bribe taking and the encouragement of toadyism and adulation, had a deleterious influence on the moral atmosphere in society.

Real care for people, for the conditions of their life and work and for social well-being, were often replaced with political flirtation – the mass distribution of awards, titles and prizes. An atmosphere of permissiveness was taking shape, and attention to detail, discipline and responsibility were declining.

Serious shortcomings in ideological and political education were in many cases disguised with ostentatious activities, and campaigns and celebrations of numerous jubilees. The world of day to day realities, and that of make-believe well-being, were increasingly diverging. The ideology and mentality of stagnation had their effect on the state of culture, literature and the arts.

(Gorbachev 1987)

Gorbachev's solution was openness and restructuring, *glasnost* and *perestroika*. His recognition of the problems of bureaucracy, cynicism, corruption, drugs and alcohol during the Brezhnev years fits well with the trends in death rates from different causes. The main causes of death which show a change in trend in the early 1970s are easily summarised (Wilkinson 1996). Homicide and purposeful injury started to rise rapidly from the mid 1970s. Mental disorders and diseases of the nervous system and sense organs had been falling but also started to rise; the same is also true of endocrine, nutritional and metabolic diseases and immunity disorders. Chronic liver disease and cirrhosis started to rise more rapidly than previously, while the rate of reduction in infectious and parasitic diseases declined substantially.

These patterns, particularly the rising deaths from homicide, chronic liver disease and cirrhosis, bear a striking resemblance to the patterns of cause-specific mortality which, as we shall see in chapter 8, are associated with a widening income distribution

(McIsaac and Wilkinson 1996). Even in the mid-1980s, the distribution of income still remained, as Atkinson has shown, rather more egalitarian than it was in Britain, but the trend in several countries (including the Soviet Union but not Czechoslovakia) was towards greater inequality (Atkinson and Mickelwright 1992a, 1992b). However, what happened to income distribution is unlikely to be the key here. Throughout Eastern Europe income differences were a less good guide to status differences than is the case in market societies. Because of the shortage of consumer goods and the necessity of extensive queuing when shopping, many people did not spend all their income. Party membership and access to special shops may have been a better guide to status, and to ownership of consumer durables, than was income itself. Indeed, in several Eastern European countries average manual wages were higher than non-manual wages (Wnuk-Lipinski and Illsley 1990). Some epidemiologists have suggested that this gave rise to problems of 'status inconsistency' which has started to creep into epidemiological literature as a possible health hazard (Siegrist et al. 1990).

It is however clear from Gorbachev's speech that there was an important deterioration in the social fabric of society. Although caused by extraneous political processes which need not have affected income differentials, the changes that took place are illuminating because, despite different causes, they share some features of social disintegration which usually accompany widening income differences elsewhere.

The Brezhnev era (1964–82) had brought a profound sense of disillusionment, especially for the older generations whose idealism and faith in the system had been partly rekindled when Khrushchev denounced the crimes and brutality of the Stalinist period. In earlier years there had been some optimism about the potential of centrally planned economies. Economic growth rates had often been better than in Western countries, which is what Khrushchev was referring to in his speech to the UN General Assembly in 1960 when he confidently predicted that the Soviet Union would 'bury' capitalism. The launching of the first satellite into space in 1957 seemed to symbolise the growing technological prowess of the Soviet Union.

However, by the 1970s that confidence had gone. Instead of believing that they were serving a socially and economically superior system, the Eastern European Communist Parties were seen increasingly as repressive agents of a foreign power, dependent on secret police and informers to maintain their power. After the crushing of the 'Prague Spring' in Czechoslovakia in 1968, Brezhnev announced what soon became known as the 'Brezhnev doctrine', saying that the Soviet Union would not remain inactive in the face of 'anti-socialist degeneration' in the Soviet bloc. This no doubt marked the beginning of a stronger Soviet influence in the political and economic life of Eastern European countries, and partly explains the similarity of their subsequent political development. The crushing of successive uprisings had publicly removed the moral claim to legitimacy of governments in Eastern Europe.

Over the years this had a devastating effect on public life. Because of the lack of pluralism and the Communist Parties' control of all institutions, people became increasingly alienated from activity in the public sphere – including work. Indeed, the cynicism with which the purge was conducted in Czechoslovakia following the crushing of the Prague Spring meant that any idealism remaining in the party was rooted out. 'Through the whole sorting operation the [Czech] Communist Party got rid of most of its active, idealistic and independently thinking members' (Simecka 1984, p. 40). The weeding-out process valued 'obedience, loyalty, dependability, mediocrity, respectability, caution [and] moral weakness' (ibid., p. 41). The corrosive effects of the regime's loss of a sense of purpose affected all areas of public life. Even values of public spiritedness were sullied with implicit support for the regime. Work and the public sphere as a whole ceased to provide opportunities for self-fulfilment and socially purposeful activity. Because of the deep sense of frustration and meaningless-ness, the family became the only area of life in which a degree of self-realisation was still possible. This is why infant mortality rates were relatively unaffected and continued to decline during the 1970s and 1980s, why women's mortality rates were less affected than men's, and why – in both sexes – the adverse trends are particularly pronounced among single people without families.

Perhaps this not only gives us some idea of the kinds of influ-ences which might account for the failure of life expectancy to increase in Eastern Europe during most of the 1970s and 1980s, but also suggests the common origins of the health trends and the uprisings of 1989. But what was the situation earlier? Why was it that, at least until 1970, countries where Communist Parties had taken power tended to have health standards so much higher than would be expected given their level of GNP per capita? Even in

1990, China, which according to the World Bank had average incomes scarcely 2 per cent of those in the USA, nevertheless achieved an average life expectancy almost equal to that of the USA in 1970.

The concept of comradeship in the state-controlled economies shares some elements with the camaraderie of wartime Britain. But at its centre is a paradox. Writing of the former Soviet Union under Stalin, Gross says that the ability of everyone to act as informers gave the arbitrary power of the state to every citizen to use against others. 'Everybody shared the power to bring down and destroy everyone else.' So important was this power that, in Gross's words, 'This ability to get anybody arrested was the great equaliser of Soviet citizens' (Gross 1982, p. 376). As well as describing the growing sense that friends could no longer be trusted, Vogel, in a paper on China, also explains the growth of a 'new ethic of comradeship' as a form of relationship between citizens. After describing the negative process of the breakdown of personal trust between people, his paper 'From friendship to comradeship: the change in personal relations in Communist China' goes on to describe the development of comradeship in more positive terms (Vogel 1965). Its essence was apparently not only in its loyalty to communism, but also its universality, in the fact that every citizen was a fellow comrade. Vogel says that 'part of the ethic underlying the concept of comrade is that there is an important way in which everyone in society is related to every other person.' 'The other side of the concept is that one should not have special relationships with certain people which would interfere with the obligations to everyone else' (ibid., p. 55). An important element in comradeship in China was 'helping other people' which, while this was apparently sometimes a euphemism for getting other people to fall into line and pull their weight, also meant a genuine willingness to spend time to help people in need. Vogel gives examples:

A student who is having trouble with his lessons should be helped by someone who can give the assistance. An old person on the street should be given assistance by someone located conveniently nearby. A newcomer to a group should be helped by someone already on hand to become acquainted with the new place, to find all the facilities that he will need. There is a positive value placed on being of assistance to others, on spending time and energy to make things easier for them. Indeed, some refugees from mainland China find it difficult to adjust in Hong Kong to the fact that no longer are people really looking after them and caring for them.

(Vogel 1965, p. 55)

Even though there is more than a suggestion that private relationships are sacrificed, it is possible that the egalitarian quality of social relations and public values played a central role in why the so-called communist countries have traditionally had higher standards of health than would be expected given their per capita income. If so, then there is at least the possibility of explaining the diminishing health performance of Eastern European countries in the 1970s and 1980s as due to a loss of an advantage they once shared with other communist countries. When Gorbachev complained of the erosion of 'lofty moral values' in the Soviet Union, of a declining 'interest in the affairs of society' and a growth in callousness and scepticism', he was surely referring to a decline in this quality of public life.

In the countries of Eastern Europe these public values were fatally identified with support for the Party and the supposedly communist project. Being a good citizen appeared as an expression of support for the government and could only be maintained where there was still a degree of idealism. As that gave way to political cynicism, the nature of public life inevitably changed.

In a paper entitled 'Social disintegration in Poland: civil society or amoral familism?', Tarkowska and Tarkowski (1991) describe the growing divide between public and private spheres of life in Poland:

> Throughout the 1970s, there was intense concern with family, friends and small social circles, in contrast to marked apathy towards public life. The politicisation of 1980–81 meant a revitalisation of the public sphere and the [brief] emergence of politics as an alternative. But with the introduction of martial law in December 1981, private life emerged supreme. . . . By 1989 a completely 'private society' had emerged.
>
> (Tarkowska and Tarkowski 1991, pp.103–4)

The psychological impact on the population of these events was demonstrated by the dramatic but temporary fall in suicides during the optimism of 1981 to which Watson drew attention (Watson 1995). After referring to the 'boycott of public life', Tarkowska and

Tarkowski say that economic shortages led to competition and antagonism between the small private social circles and tended in turn to create 'aggression, social pathology and all the features of an "unfriendly society" ... divided between "family members" and "strangers"' (Tarkowska and Tarkowski 1991, p. 104). It is particularly interesting that to describe the degeneration of Polish society during this period, the authors draw explicitly on the concept of 'amoral familism' which Banfield used to characterise the areas of southern Italy later found by Putnam to have the lowest levels of civic development (Banfield 1958).

One of the most interesting things about the widening health gap between Eastern and Western Europe during the 1970s and 1980s was discovered by Leon (D. Leon, personal communication, 1996). For each cause of death – cancers of each site, stroke, heart disease, infections, etc. – he calculated the ratio of death rates in Eastern and Western Europe. He then did the same for the ratio of death rates between lower and upper social classes in Britain. He found that there was a correlation between the two of about 0.7 – slightly more for men and slightly less for women. In other words, the causes of death which had the highest excess in Eastern compared to Western Europe tended to be the same causes as had the highest excess in lower compared to higher social classes in Britain. Some causes, like breast cancer, did not contribute to either gradient. Because the same causes were elevated in each comparison, it suggests that they were the expression of similar environmental influences.

JAPAN

The fifth and last example of where these issues come together in an informative way is in Japan. As we have already seen, Japanese life expectancy has increased dramatically during the last few decades as its income differences have narrowed (Marmot and Davey Smith 1989; Wilkinson 1992). As recently as 1970 it was much like Britain in both respects (Wilkinson 1986). By the end of the 1980s it had the highest life expectancy in the world and the narrowest income differentials of any country reporting to the World Bank.

The decline in income inequality which has marked much of the development of Japanese society in the postwar period reflects the special development of Japanese capitalism during and after the Second World War. Dore describes the operation of Japanese capitalism before the war as differing little from the pattern established in other countries. But reform of Japanese industry and society was enabled by the extent to which the power and position of the Japanese establishment was weakened and discredited by the military defeat. Immediately after the war 'all who held formal authority in all spheres of Japanese life, including industry, were demoralized and no longer confident of their power to command' (Dore 1973, p. 115). 'Exhortations to loyalty and service gave way to the propaganda of democracy, equality, liberty and individual dignity' (ibid., p. 116). Dore refers to 'the great post-1945 flood of egalitarian ideas' (ibid., p.339) and says 'Japanese industry has had, whereas British industry has not, its social democratic revolution' (ibid., p. 115). In addition, the American occupation meant that postwar reconstruction was strongly influenced by the advice of American experts who had no personal vested interests or loyalty to the old establishment.

However, some of the most important changes were a response to the war itself. As part of the wartime mobilization of the Japanese economy, the government took 'draconian' powers over industry (Dore 1995). These included the requirement that new members of companies' boards of directors could only be appointed with government approval and must have knowledge and/or experience of the industry concerned. The result was that the proportion of company directors who had worked their way up through the company rose during the war from around one-third in the mid-1930s to over 95 per cent in 1949 (Dore 1996; Aoki and Dore 1994). This, in conjunction with several fundamental labour reforms immediately after the war, provided a different social basis for the development of the Japanese working environment. Provisions which enabled trade union leaders to gain experience at board level have resulted in some of the largest companies now being run by former union leaders.

In his important analysis of the differences between the social organisation of two Hitachi factories in Japan and two English Electric plants, Dore gives 'considerable weight to an increasingly general desire for social equality' in Japan (Dore 1973, p. 11). He describes how this led, not so much to the disappearance of hierarchy, but to a different kind of hierarchy.

The contrast . . . is between a class system and a system of infinitely divisible strata. English Electric employees have a conception of the status system of their factory – and, for that matter of their society – in terms of a few more or less homogeneous layers separated by marked gaps. The extent to which people are conscious of the gaps depends on the *variety* of differentiating criteria which *coincide* on the same lines of division – income, method of payment, toilets, canteens, holidays, pension rights, dress, accent, union membership, etc. – in addition to functional authority positions. In the Hitachi system, by contrast, there are far fewer discontinuities – toilets, canteens, etc. do not demarcate status groups. Pay scales are a *single* continuum.

(Dore 1973, p.258)

Even where such discontinuities do exist, they not only fail to coincide with each other, but may actually cross-cut each other.

The different experiences of social stratification also seem to show up in surveys that suggest not only that many more Japanese have difficulty in assigning themselves to a social class than do the English, but that support for Japanese political parties is less polarised by social class.

Within the firm, 'Hitachi directors have nearly all graduated to their position after a lifetime of work in the firm . . . Hitachi directors are more likely to see themselves as elders of a corporate community rather than as men responsible to the shareholders for wringing the maximum profit out of the shareholders property, the firm' (ibid., p. 260). 'In terms of dignity, or prestige status, Hitachi workers are less deprived than their English Electric counterparts' (ibid., p. 259). 'Hitachi's concern with the group, its integration and its collective performance, runs right down to the shop-floor work team' (ibid., p. 231). 'Japan was and still largely is a "groupish" society. That is why a system which minimizes rivalry and maximises co-operation and security . . . can be more easily directed to co-operative efforts in pursuit of the ends of the group as a whole' (ibid., pp. 230–1).

The 'groupishness' of society is closely related to what is often seen as the paternalism of Japanese industry. The emphasis on loyalty, group membership and performance is fostered partly by systems of group targets and bonuses, but also by the much more extensive social roles which Japanese foremen have compared to their Western counterparts. As well as being responsible for a wider range of social activities at work, such as celebrations, outings and parties, they are also expected to have a detailed knowledge of the families of workers in their group and may take an active part in their family affairs.

Over most of the postwar period, Japanese income differentials seem to have diminished and are now considerably smaller than in other Western countries and very much smaller than they are in Britain or the United States. In addition, the success of the Japanese economy has made it easier not only to avoid lay-offs in recessions, but also to provide more job security and to keep unemployment levels down. However, the different approach of senior managers and directors in Japanese firms to safeguarding people's positions shows that there are also important differences in morality. It has been a common expectation that senior managers would take self-imposed pay cuts in hard times rather than lay off shop-floor workers (Dore 1995).

Some of the same basic contrasts between Japanese and Western society were clearly visible in a comparison of Japanese and American policing methods (Bayley 1976). We shall discuss these in chapter 8 in the context of the long-term decline in Japanese crime rates which have accompanied the dramatic improvements in health and the narrowing income differences. Bayley makes it quite clear that the Japanese police are not merely law enforcers but also have a mandate to act as moral teachers. He says that character is regarded as responsive to social pressures and offenders are expected to accept the community's terms for resocialisation with the aim that they will feel a moral obligation to assist actively in preserving the moral consensus in the community (Bayley 1976). A bizarre indication of the power of the explicitly social mediation of life was provided in a recent newspaper story of two gang members who called into a police station to apologise for the murder of a policeman mistaken for a member of another gang (Andrews 1995).

What is important about the Japanese example in the present context is neither the idealisation of a society less wracked by class divisions, nor the fears of the sacrifice of individuality to a system which may appear to use paternalism to serve the interests of capital. It is instead the association of a narrow income distribution with a public sphere of life which has a real social content. Instead of a moral and social vacuum mediated only by market relationships, life beyond the family has a well-developed *social* structure. Almost regardless of the ideological uses to which it might be put, public life is explicitly part of social life. While it used to be thought that some of the distinctive characteristics of Japanese society were merely remnants of its recent agricultural past which would disappear in the course of economic development, it is clear that the social framework has instead contained some of the anti-social features of market society which might have threatened it.

CONCLUSION

It is clear that wider and narrower income differences are associated with important differences in the social fabric of society. These examples have provided more than cross-sectional evidence. Britain during the two world wars showed more rapid improvements in health as the country became more cohesive and egalitarian. The example of Roseto showed the loss of the town's health advantage as its social cohesion declined. The Eastern Europe experience showed the loss of a health advantage that communist countries had previously shared with more egalitarian societies. It also showed that this loss was associated particularly with the growing meaninglessness and decay of life in the public sphere. Finally, in Japan it is possible to see the more rapid improvement in life expectancy as inequalities were reduced. In all these examples we see an association between egalitarianism, social cohesion and better health. However, rather than putting together a neatly packaged set of conclusions from these examples, their purpose has been to raise some of the wider sociological and structural issues in a practical context rather than in a purely theoretical discussion. The examples illustrate a variety of backward and forward linkages between income distribution and characteristics of social, ideological, business and economic life.

Although we can see in each example that there are these wider connections, it is not clear in which direction causality goes. Perhaps it can go in both directions. Although a narrower income distribution leads to a more egalitarian social ethic, it also looks as if exogenous factors which create a more egalitarian ethic tend also to lead to narrowing income differences. If a more egalitarian social ethos were to develop exogenously, for reasons unrelated to income distribution, it is implausible that such a society would tolerate great material inequalities without making efforts to reduce them. It is also unlikely that its cohesiveness would last if it did not reduce inequality. If, on the other hand, there were exogenous changes in income distribution, the evidence from a variety of sources suggests that they would quickly bring about changes in the sense of social cohesion or division. So however cohesive societies are formed, a narrow distribution of income is a necessary condition for their survival and is likely to serve as a marker for important characteristics of the social fabric.

Despite the mixed evidence in these examples on the direction of causality, it might be thought that the widening of income differentials which overtook a number of countries during the 1980s (the effects in Britain were discussed in the previous chapter) was a clear example of an exogenous change in income distribution which led to a deterioration in the social fabric of society. However, even here the evidence is ambiguous. Those who would say that the growth in income inequality came first would point to its source in international competition and new technology which weakened the market position of people with low levels of skill and education. In contrast others might argue that monetarism as an economic ideology came first, and that it always had the covert aim of weakening the bargaining power of labour and cutting back the welfare state in the hope of using increased income differentials to stimulate economic growth.

The fact that income distribution and the quality of a society's social fabric are so closely linked perhaps means that it is futile to try to establish an order of determination. There is a constant interaction between the two, not from one year or period of years to another which would make it meaningful to try to establish a direction of causality, or even from one month to another, but a day by day interaction. The interaction between social and economic processes takes place continuously throughout society with the occasional shifts one way or the other in the combined centre of gravity.

Social cohesion and a sense of community are important themes running through all these examples. Though the more egalitarian and cohesive structure of societies with narrower income differences has, in these examples, often been fostered (or co-opted) to serve some ulterior purpose such as the war effort in Britain, economic growth in Japan or support for the communist parties in Eastern Europe, Roseto and the Italian regions show that this need not be so. But it is also clear that greater egalitarianism has benefited health whether or not it has served other ideological purposes. If one were to pick out something close to the heart of the difference between more and less egalitarian societies, it would surely be something to do with the social nature of public life. Instead of merely market or self-interested relations between families or households, it appears that in more egalitarian societies the public sphere of life remains a more social sphere than it does elsewhere. It remains dominated by people's involvement in the social, ethical and human life of the society, rather than being abandoned to market values and transactions. People come together to pursue and contribute to broader, shared social purposes: that is the social cohesion. That these forces are fostered to serve the war effort or higher productivity is an indication of the extent to which the breakdown of social cohesion weakens not just a society's health, but also its productive efforts.

Since I wrote this chapter, new evidence has been produced showing that social cohesion is very closely related to income distribution among the states of the United States. In a most important paper called 'Social capital, income inequality and mortality' to be published in the *American Journal of Public Health*, Kawachi, Kennedy and their colleagues provide quantitative evidence that social cohesion provides the link between income distribution and mortality in the USA. This finding is doubly important: it not only provides the first quantitative evidence (as opposed to the qualitative evidence above) that social cohesion mediates between income distribution and mortality, but it also confirms on US data what Putnam reports but disregards in Italy, that social cohesion is very strongly related to income distribution. This is a message no politician should be allowed to ignore.

Chapter 7

An anthropology of social cohesion

From a historical perspective, modern societies are still feeling their way towards a satisfactory social organisation of the highly integrated productive system which economic development has so recently produced. With few exceptions it was – even in most developed countries – only a few generations ago that the world consisted predominantly of small farmers producing largely for their own consumption without more than a marginal involvement in commerce. In Britain, where industrialisation first appeared, it is only necessary to go back to my grandmother's grandmother to reach someone born before the first spate of railway building, before the first fruits of the Industrial Revolution. In Japan it has been estimated that as recently as the 1860s only some 5 per cent of the population were engaged in any kind of wage employment (Dore 1973). The monetary economy, rather than being a permanent feature of human society, has only become the dominant force in the lives of most of the world's population during the last half century. Although money has a long history, it played only a marginal role in the lives of self-sufficient peasant producers. Even the role which money did have in pre-industrial societies was often tightly constrained – with prices and wages fixed by tradition or even law, and clear prohibitions on usury.

When we look forwards rather than backwards into the past, it is clear that the way money works and is used is going to change beyond recognition as it becomes increasingly electronic. If physical coinage and notes actually disappear and the flow of income and expenditure for every member of society is something registered only in the memories of central computers, it is likely that money will develop a different meaning. Rather than having cash in your pocket or not having it, people's expenditure is already increasingly limited more by abstract constructs like their credit rating. Despite both the sense of the overwhelming power of the market economy as it completely saturates modern life and of the apparent inevitability of its dominance of human affairs, it is important to remember how recent this power is and how rapidly it is changing. As societies search out a more social *modus vivendi* with the modern interdependent productive system, it is important that we see the problems while remembering how recent the dominance of the cash economy is, and just how fast it is changing.

Income differentials have become the most powerful expression and determinant of social and economic inequality but inequality can have other bases. Slavery, hereditary positions and titles, feudal and cast systems all institutionalise inequality in different forms. With the rise of the cash economy more and more of the social, categorical and situational markers of status have given way to monetary ones. The modern effects of income inequality are the combined effects of inequality and the market. However, for most of human existence human societies were held together by a very different form of exchange.

GIFT EXCHANGE

In many early forms of society, particularly hunters and gatherers, herders and slash-and-burn agriculturalists, food sharing and gift exchange prevailed throughout the nomadic group, village or tribe. Social anthropologists have devoted a great deal of attention to trying to understand the way different kinds of goods were exchanged, the patterns of food sharing, gift giving and the norms of reciprocity. Food sharing and gift exchange were almost always the dominant form of distribution within early societies.

However, gift giving was often not confined just to exchange within the community but was used more widely to include exchange with neighbouring groups of people sometimes on a more ritualised basis. Even when goods were regularly exchanged with other communities to fulfil the economic function of supplying each with things they could not easily provide for themselves, the exchange often took the form of gift exchange and was carried out by long-established 'trade partners', between whom negative reciprocity was suppressed and haggling outlawed.

Most societies showed a strong taboo on any open expressions of material self-interest. 'The !Kung do not trade amongst themselves.

They consider the procedure undignified and avoid it because it is too likely to stir up bad feelings' (Marshall 1961, p. 242 as quoted in Sahlins 1974, p. 232). Discussing the self-interested inland trade which takes place between unrelated tribes in Polynesia, Hogbin said, 'The parties seem slightly ashamed . . . and conclude their arrangements outside the village. Commerce, it is considered, should be carried on away from where people live, preferably alongside the road or the beach' (as quoted by Sahlins 1974, p. 236).

Where forms of primitive money were used even within a society and there was competition for scarce resources, it was almost always confined to competition for luxury or ceremonial goods: food and other necessities were still shared equally (Nash 1966). No doubt an important part of why food sharing was so predominant and why social systems avoided competition for access to essentials was to remove a source of conflict. The social conflict resulting from individuals or groups barring each other from access to essentials has to be avoided at all costs. As Firth points out, the results of the Maori system of food distribution was that 'starvation or real want in one family was impossible while others in the village were abundantly supplied with food' (Firth 1959, p. 290). Quotes such as these are commonplace. Schapera (1930, p. 148 as quoted in Sahlins 1974, p. 264) said of the Bushmen: 'Food . . . is private property and belongs to the person who has obtained it. Everyone who has food is, however, expected to give to all those who have none. The result is that practically all food obtained is evenly distributed through the whole camp.' Radcliffe-Brown used almost identical words to describe the system of food sharing among the Andaman Islanders (Radcliffe-Brown 1948, p. 43 as quoted in Sahlins 1974, p. 264).

In two important essays drawing on a vast anthropological literature on early exchange systems, Sahlins developed this analysis of systems of gift exchange further (Sahlins 1974). He explained the predominance of gift exchange and food sharing in primitive societies as a way of keeping the peace. Leaning on Hobbes's political philosophy, he describes early forms of society as having the potential for conflict, of 'warre of everyone against everyone'. It is not that there is actual war in a Hobbesian 'state of nature' but, in the absence of an overriding power (a sovereign or 'common power to keep them all in awe') capable of preventing conflict, it is up to each individual to conduct their relations with others in a way designed to keep the peace and avoid animosity. In other words, where there is no police force you are obliged to make your own peace with people. And gift exchange and food sharing is how it was done.

Sahlins notes that there is a continuum of sociability in gift giving and forms of exchange. It runs all the way from 'sacrifice in favour of another to self-interested gain at the expense of another'. At one end is the unreciprocated gift, in the middle are various forms of reciprocal gift exchange with looser or tighter norms about the timing and nature of the reciprocal gift, and at the other end are various forms of openly self-interested market exchange and haggling. He emphasises the moral element in gift exchange quoting from ethnographies of different societies: 'the feeling was present that to trade for food was reprehensible' (Sahlins 1974, p. 218). 'Whatever the utilitarian value [of reciprocal gift exchange], and there need be none, there is always a moral purpose ... to provide a friendly feeling ... and unless it did this it failed its purpose' (ibid., p. 220). 'The striking of equivalence [in reciprocal gift exchange] ... is a demonstrable foregoing of self-interest on each side, some renunciation of hostile intent or of indifference in favour of mutuality' (ibid., p. 220).

The gift, which brings with it a sense of indebtedness and an obligation to reciprocate, amounts, in Sahlins' eyes, to a primitive social contract: it is, as he says, the way people 'come to terms' with one another. In all human societies, receiving a gift creates a sense of indebtedness and an obligation to reciprocate. Indeed, this seems to be one of the few universals of human society. It is a social bond: 'if friends make gifts, gifts make friends' (ibid., p. 186). So powerful is the sense of indebtedness that it was often the basis of chiefly power. Those who give most would also gain most influence and power by making people indebted to them.

Sahlins concludes his paper with the words:

> Here has been given a discourse on economics in which 'econo-mizing' appears mainly as an exogenous factor. The organizing principles of economy have been sought elsewhere. To the extent that they have been found outside man's presumed hedonist propensity, a strategy of primitive economics is suggested that is something the reverse of economic orthodoxy.
>
> (ibid., p. 230)

The implication is that in these societies the maintenance of good social relations was more important than narrower material considerations.

These institutional practices are important not simply because they provide a contrast with the prevailing exchange systems today, but because they represent cultural patterns which evolved independently among different societies all over the world and endured, not for an odd century or so, but for hundreds of thousands of years – covering the vast majority of human existence. They reflect the forms through which human social life was organized and the institutions through which people came to know themselves, their behaviour and their relations with others.

The way that behaviour is institutionally structured will give us radically different views as to how we are related to one another and what we understand and experience as the 'normal' or 'natural' relationship between people. Whether actions are in fact self-interested at some other level is perhaps not the point. What matters is whether the cultural forms we use proclaim self-interest or mutuality as the norm in human relations.

The exchange systems through which we are brought together as individuals in society not only build into us powerful assumptions about how we are related to one another but also appear to tell us how social or self-interested our basic nature is. Inevitably, we experience the institutionalised pattern of material relations through which we live our lives as if they were a direct expression of our inner nature and relatedness to one another.

Sahlins' use of Hobbes's political philosophy has striking implications which Sahlins does not develop. Given the absence of any overriding governmental power, we should – as Sahlins suggests – see gift exchange, food sharing and the materially egalitarian nature of early societies as the result of people's need to keep the peace themselves. If he is right, then the converse should also be right: the overt self-interest of market transactions and great material inequality of modern hierarchical societies is predicated on the presence of an overriding authority capable of keeping the peace. The police, courts and prisons not only absolve people of the need to maintain peace themselves but enable us all to live in a way that could cause conflict. We can conduct our affairs in ways that are not conducive to social harmony because we are protected from most of the social consequences of doing so. Material inequality and market relations are so incongruous with caring and harmonious social relations that an overriding governmental power capable of maintaining social order is a necessity. Only under its jurisdiction can the complaints of the dispossessed be safely ignored.

Powerful social taboos against open expressions of material self-interest in exchange systems were not confined to the earliest forms of society. During the transition of peasant class societies to the market – long after the loss of primitive egalitarianism – the historical transition to a fully commercial society was marked by a major upheaval of moral attitudes. Perhaps the most famous contribution to this moral change was Bernard Mandeville's *Fable of the bees: or private vices, publick benefits*, which was first published in 1714. Widely regarded as having paved the way for a more commercial or capitalist ethic, Mandeville proposed what seemed to many the morally offensive idea that the pursuit of private self-interest was beneficial to society at large (Goldsmith 1985). *The Fable of the bees* 'involved a rejection of the prevalent political and social ideology and offered a different social theory ... [which] was peculiarly suited to justifying a ... commercial, or ... capitalist, society' (Goldsmith 1985, p. 123). 'Human society would be improved by people whose actions were selfishly directed to seeking pleasure' (ibid., p. 162). The central issue was a change from a morality expressed in the earlier view that the more the most privileged sections of society consumed, the less there would be left for everyone else, to the new view that increased consumption by the rich was beneficial to society because it provided the poor with work and earnings. One reflected the nature of agricultural production and the limited supply of land, while the other reflected a commercial society in which people seemed – almost literally – to live on money by selling their labour. In contrast to those who blamed society's problems on the unmoderated love of luxury and riches which appeared as part of the debauchery and corruption of the wealthy, Mandeville proclaimed in his satirical style that luxury 'employ'd a million of the poor'. Even theft kept locksmiths in business. The argument caused widespread outrage and continued to be controversial throughout the eighteenth century. Amongst others, both David Hume and Adam Smith were contributors to the debate. Despite the elements of a monetised economy in earlier centuries, monetary exchange had been regulated to keep the expression of self-interest within socially prescribed bounds. In medieval society wages and prices of important commodities were fixed by law and tradition at levels thought just or fair. There was not a free market and it was illegal to profit from temporary shortages.

The development of the new economic morality went hand in

hand with what is sometimes dubbed the 'commercial revolution' or the 'birth of consumer society' which took place in eighteenth-century England (McKendrick *et al.* 1982). The period was marked by the growth of conspicuous consumption, the rise of fashion, and the development of shopping and commercial life. It was at the end of the eighteenth century that Napoleon referred to England as 'a nation of shopkeepers'.

In the same period financial interests also became a recognisable force in society. The Bank of England had been founded in 1694 and there was a growing stock market. The growth of the market as the ruling principle of economic life clearly required the abandonment of earlier moral sensibilities. One of the market's major advantages was to function as an apparently entirely mechanistic and impersonal distributor of its injustices. It absolved the privileged and powerful from their social responsibilities and ensured that the poor could rarely blame anyone in particular for their plight. The idea that the market could miraculously transform the unrestrained pursuit of self-interest into an act of kindness to one's fellow human beings clearly had natural allies in several sections of society.

The degree of inequality in modern societies shows the extent to which we ignore each other's welfare. In countries where some go hungry while others live well, the divisions are harder and cruder than they are in states where social security systems ensure that people have at least a minimum subsistence. Instead of giving separate messages, the social meanings implied by inequality and the market come together. If the social environment in which the open separation, or opposition of interests, expressed in market transactions and in the dependency of households on separate incomes, is one of relative material equality, its divisive social meanings are greatly softened. In effect, the divisive meanings of the market become stronger or weaker according to how wide or narrow income differences are. Where they are wider, the principles of the market tend to overflow into areas of social life. Market societies are transmuted into market economies as the principles of social organisation are subordinated to the logic of private gain.

There are a number of psychological processes which increase the tolerance of social injustice and give an appearance of legitimacy to the material inequality to which the market gives rise. In particular there is a strong tendency for people to assume that their position in society is a reflection of their innate worth. In *The hidden injuries of class*, Sennett and Cobb (1973) showed that among manual workers in Boston the most profound effect of their relatively lowly position was their belief that they were inherently less capable than those above them. Either people accept that their position is a reflection of their ability or they engage in a constant struggle to improve their standing and save their self-esteem.

Numerous psychological studies have shown that we all have a tendency to infer ability from the social trappings of office – even in situations where there can clearly be no possible justification for doing so. In one experiment participants taken in pairs were randomly given the roles of playing 'questioners' or 'contestants' (Ross 1978). The questioners had to use their own general knowledge to think up challenging general knowledge questions to which they knew the answers, and then to put them to their contestant partners. The questioners, their contestant partners and a group of observers all knew that their roles had been randomly allocated. Yet at the end of the session it was found that all three groups – questioners, contestants and observers – rated the general knowledge of the questioners significantly higher than that of the contestants. Indeed, on a scale of 1–100, the contestants rated their own general knowledge as only 40 and that of their questioner partners as 65. Similar evidence shows that we infer from our own and others' roles in an institution or position in society to an opinion of our relative abilities. The other side of this coin is the effect which status differences can have on people's self-esteem and confidence.

An important aspect of the market and wage labour is the individualism which it institutionalises. At the centre of the concept of individualism is the practical separation of each person's interests and identity from those of others. Indeed, individualism is most fundamentally expressed by the role of cash in a market economy as we earn and spend our 'living', opposed as buyers and sellers in the marketplace. Dependent on individual incomes, my income is for my needs and any acknowledgement of your needs endangers the sufficiency of my income and so of my security.

The economic necessity of earning and spending, and the economic institutions through which we do that, contains a rationality which animates a large part of our lives. This logic of possessive individualism which grows out of the opposition of marketised 'interests' provides economists with their rational choice theory.

But instead of that logic remaining simply an external fact of life, it becomes internalised. Instead of seeing the real situational sources of our behaviour, it has become clear that we infer an inner rationality as if it were inherent within us. We experience ourselves as endowed with the appropriate social, material and acquisitive internal dispositions and motivations, which our actions seem to express. As a result the self-interested individualism of the marketplace spills over into other areas of social life. If we come to know ourselves through the market, then we behave as if its motivations were inherent deep within us. The nature of public life changes and human interaction becomes dominated by the asocial values of the market.

Social psychology has demonstrated the extent to which we come to understand ourselves, to infer our nature and characteristics, not from a genuinely internal introspective source, but as observers of our behaviour. To an extraordinary extent we use situational and behavioural clues to interpret not only our own emotions and motivations, but also to infer those of others. We come to believe that human beings are by nature what their culture suggests they are. Thus, if we live through institutions that have an opposition of interests as their rationality, then this is the way we will read human nature. This is why, throughout history, from one kind of society to another, people have believed that the institutions of their particular society are merely human nature writ large. People in societies where gift exchange was the norm grew up with one set of assumptions about how they were related to one another; we grow up with a different set.

The human tendency to make this inference has the additional effect that we underestimate the scope for change. It makes all the flaws in society appear as if they arose from the inadequacies of human beings rather than from the inadequacies of institutions. This inversion is so strong that it serves to stabilise the cultural forms through which we live. By the same token, we fail to realise how soon a different social order might come to seem a reflection of a different human nature.

Much of the experimental work on our perception of our emotions and inner motivational world was stimulated by evidence which seemed to show that different emotions were accompanied by broadly similar states of physiological arousal (Kleinke 1978). Instead of an introspective process by which we reach into an inner source to experience the truth of what we are feeling, it was found that emotions were distinguished from each other largely by cognitive processes involving an interpretation of our situation. The emotional experience of a given state of physiological arousal was found to depend on the perception of situational clues. To demonstrate the cognitive and situational contribution to the experience of an emotion depended on manipulating the situation of experimental subjects so as to induce them to 'misattribute' their state of arousal from its initial cognitive source. Given some deceptive experimental manipulation of the environment, it was shown that physical arousal caused initially by fear, by humour or annoyance, by adrenaline injections or even by exercise, could be experienced as quite a different emotion and then give rise to behaviour expressive of a different emotion. This experiential process of misattribution did not depend on any verbal expression, conscious recall or interrogation.

One of the less startling examples which is nevertheless relevant to the market, concerns the effect of payment on intrinsic and extrinsic motivation. Two separate groups of students were asked to work on a series of puzzles (Deci 1971). One group was told they would be paid a fixed sum of money for every correct solution, while the other group was paid nothing. After one hour both groups were given a rest period during which they were secretly watched. The prediction that the students who were not paid would regard themselves as intrinsically motivated and would be more likely to continue working during the rest period was confirmed. This suggests that the perception of liking or disliking doing the puzzles was not wholly determined by any internal knowledge of how enjoyable or unpleasant the experience of working on them had been, but was significantly influenced by a situational clue as to their motivation.

Another frequently replicated experiment illustrating the same basic point is called the 'forbidden toy' experiment. It involves asking children not to play with a particular toy while an adult supervisor is temporarily absent (Kleinke 1978). One group is given a mild warning not to disobey while the other is given a much more severe warning. In the event, the children are watched and it is found that none plays with the forbidden toy. When assessed later, the evidence shows that the children who had been given a severe warning have come to find the toy more attractive than those given a mild warning. Given that there are several possible interpretations of this result, the experiment has been repeated with a number of variations. The results have shown that children given a mild warning are more likely to infer that they did not play with the toy because they did not find it very attractive. The ones given a severe threat are less likely to experience themselves as having acted freely when they did not play with it, and so do not infer any personal lack of interest in it as an explanation for leaving it alone.

This is now a well-developed field of experimental social psychology with a body of theory resulting from a large number of quite different kinds of experiments showing how labile are even strong emotions of anger, fear, disgust and attraction. In each case we find that the nature of an emotion is not simply the experience of an introspective internal touchstone, but is inferred from a cognitive construction of the situation.

This work is important in the present context because it demonstrates that with little genuinely internal knowledge of our motivations and feelings, we read our internal nature from our external behaviour in a particular socially structured context. As Bem says, 'individuals come to "know" their own attitudes, emotions and other internal states partially by inferring them from observations of their own overt behaviour and/or the circumstances in which this behavior occurs' (Bem 1972, p. 5). Essentially, self-perception is a product of beliefs about the causes of behaviour and, because of the weakness of genuinely introspective sources of self-awareness, has much in common with our perception of each other. We read what we take to be the inner world from socially and institutionally motivated and structured external behaviour. However, in our conscious understanding we assume the process works the other way round. Indeed, the tendency – mentioned earlier – to see social institutions as if they were expressions of human nature seems to be supported by what has been called 'the fundamental attribution error'. This is a systematic tendency noted by social psychologists for people to underestimate the impact of external situational factors and to overestimate the role of internal motivating dispositions in their perception of other people's behaviour (Ross, L. 1978). In other words, instead of seeing the real constraints of the situation, behaviour is perceived as if it were simply an expression of an inbuilt disposition. So sensitive is people's behaviour to their situation that it has been possible to show that many supposed psychological characteristics – which were thought to be permanent personality characteristics – show little or no cross-situational stability (Mischel 1986). Sometimes the experimental manipulation of very subtle situational inputs was enough to overwhelm interpersonal differences in what had been regarded as relatively stable personality traits.

It is important to recognise that this work is not referring simply to people's conscious recall or self-reports of their feelings or motivations. Instead, it deals with how people's behaviour seems to be shaped by perceptions of their feelings which, rather than coming from any genuine internal source, appear to be no more than a plausible cognitive inference of what they would be likely to feel in that situation.

A particularly clear indicator of the strength of the influence which the market has on social relations is the way its extent coincides with the boundaries of the family. The boundaries of the family coincide with the transition from market relations to sharing. When we talk about a society as having an extended family system, what it means in practice is that a wider circle of relations have a call on one another's resources and a duty towards one another's material welfare. In general, families and household members live on a shared household income: even if not all income is shared, food and household facilities are. When a couple get married or start living together, an important part of that is the sharing of expenses and taking mutual responsibility for each other's welfare. When speaking of wider kinship networks in primitive societies, E.B. Tylor pointed out that kindred goes with kindness, 'two words whose common derivation expresses . . . one of the main principles of social life' (as quoted in Sahlins 1974, p. 196). It would be interesting to know how far the perception of different social and emotional relatedness results from the way the economic arrangements create or destroy a common identity of interests, and how much the economic arrangements follow prior emotional ties.

As well as practising gift exchange, pre-agricultural human societies were highly egalitarian. Indeed for the vast majority of prehistory (perhaps around 2.5 million years) our gathering and hunting forebears lived in small egalitarian groups. Anthropologists have drawn attention to a number of different factors as the basis for this egalitarianism. Sahlins' explanation of the systems of gift exchange and food sharing was, by implication, also an explanation of the material egalitarianism of early forms of society (Sahlins 1974). Both were ways of keeping the peace between individuals in the absence of any external Hobbesian force which would do it for them.

Other anthropologists have produced different explanations of the egalitarianism of early societies. Woodburn has characterised the highly egalitarian societies of gatherers and hunters as having what he calls 'immediate return' economies rather than 'delayed return' economies (Woodburn 1982). The difference is the extent to which food production involves delay between the application of labour and the resulting product. All agriculture obviously involves delayed return, whereas foraging for what grows naturally requires little or no delay between the effort of collection and consumption. Where sophisticated tools are involved, there is also a delay between the application of the labour needed to make them and the resulting consumables they help to produce. These forms of delay lead to property rights linking those who applied the labour to the final product. In Woodburn's view, even these early forms of property lead to a departure from the most egalitarian forms of social organisation.

In contrast to both these views, Goody analysed the growth of powers of coercion (Goody 1971). He suggested that how hierarchical or egalitarian societies are depends as much upon control over the means of destruction as it does on control of the means of production. Some weapons – like stone tools, spears, bows and arrows – are essentially democratic in that anyone can make them and it is difficult to deny people access to them. On the other hand, guns can only be obtained from other sources, and if people manage to gain a monopoly in access to them (or to any other superior weaponry), they have the power to coerce others. Clearly the means of production are also important. Class systems depend on controlling access to the means of production in ways that necessarily differ at different stages of development. The strategy of controlling labour will differ according to the ease of gaining independent access to productive resources (Wilkinson 1973).

Clearly these four views are compatible with one another, though their relevance will differ from one kind of society to another and from one stage of development to another. They are all compatible with the view that social harmony was of paramount importance in early societies and involved avoiding the threats to it which arise from conflict for scarce resources. In a book with the health effects of inequality at its core, it is important to recognise that throughout most of human history and prehistory, human societies have made a point of avoiding some of the economic causes of social disharmony and have preferred more egalitarian social systems. The fact that we have had, throughout most of the existence of our species, what is by modern standards a remarkably egalitarian mode of social organisation, suggests that we may not be psychologically well adapted to inequality and individualism. The effect of inequality and subordinate status on survival could be seen as a confirmation of this. While the short-term stress responses which prepare the body for action clearly have fundamentally important survival advantages, the effects of chronic stress, which is a frequent concomitant of low social status and the lack of mutually supportive social relations, appears to be something our bodies are not used to (chapter 10).

From time to time people ignore the evidence that we are psychologically adapted to living in groups with more egalitarian social relations and cite hierarchy among chimps as our closest primate relatives to suggest that inequality is innate in humans. However, in a book called *The egalitarians*, Power (1991) argues that chimpanzees only departed from an egalitarian social organisation when artificial feeding was introduced.

Because it is so difficult to study wild chimps when you have to follow them around as they roam freely, observers started to feed them so that they would stay close to observation posts. They arranged a system of regular feeding from boxes which could be opened remotely at set times. Power argues that this precipitated fundamental changes in social organisation (Power 1991). She points to the very different accounts of chimp social organisation and behaviour before and after artificial feeding became the usual way of observing the animals in the wild. Regular feeding times led to large numbers of animals congregating and waiting tensely for the boxes of bananas to be opened. Quarrels and fighting broke out. Power says:

> The impact upon apes of the human controlled, totally unnatural feeding situations, was grave in terms of the effect upon behavior, societal tone and relationships. Under the tension of waiting with others for the fruit ... the chimpanzees became fiercely, directly competitive; and the radical change which proved devastating to the whole adapted social order began.
>
> (Power 1991, p.70)

Distributional patterns were disrupted and neighbouring groups became more hostile to one another. Territorial behaviour 'shifted away from the relatively peaceful, ritualized territoriality typical of nonhuman animals, towards a more aggressive and violent type of behaviour' (Goodall 1986, p. 528 as quoted in Power 1991, p. 73).

Relations within groups also changed dramatically. Observers who reported seeing only one brief conflict between chimps in two years before artificial feeding, reported 284 cases after feeding was introduced, of which 60 per cent took place as a direct result of the feeding. Gradually a clear social hierarchy, based on aggressive displays, threats of violence or actual violence, developed. One observer is quoted as saying that it was typically the animals which were most insecure and most in need of status who were most likely to behave aggressively and so gain hierarchical status.

Not only social, but also sexual relations underwent fundamental changes. The autonomous sexual choice of wild chimps of both sexes, which had prevailed before artificial feeding, was gradually replaced by coercive male pressure on oestrus females. Power's account of the earlier pattern would sound implausible if it were not so well documented. She describes 'a complete absence of any sign of exclusive rights of males to estrous females and no competition for access, no attempt to monopolize them sexually, no permanent sexual partners and no signs of possessiveness or aggression between males in this, or indeed any other, situation' (Power 1991, p. 77). But after the changes in social structure following the introduction of feeding, mating patterns which had seemed to serve wider social functions were replaced by more exclusive, competitive and possessive patterns.

Discussing how leadership fits into an egalitarian human context, Power (1991) generalises from a number of anthropological sources. She says that a leadership role in different activities is usually simply an acknowledgement of someone's particular knowledge or skill in that area. She says: 'The leader role is not sought after, and those who are in the role change constantly, as needs and circumstances change. The role is spontaneously assigned by the group, conferred on some member in some particular situation, not taken or seized by an individual' (ibid., p. 47).

Leadership is persuasive, not authoritarian, and serves only to guide the band towards the consensus that is the real locus of decision. Therefore others' autonomy and self-reliance are not diminished by dependence on the authority of any central or prestige figure. There is no loss or gain of self-esteem through taking either leader or follower role. The emphasis in these societies is on generalized mutuality.

(ibid., p. 47)

The fact that chimpanzee social organisation is not always competitive and hierarchical, means that reports of pecking orders and social hierarchies among animals cannot be used to suggest that social hierarchy in human societies has a 'natural' or genetic basis. Clearly even among non-human primates, different forms of social organisation are possible and we may be wrong to think of social hierarchies as typical among our closest relatives.

Chapter 8

The symptoms of disintegration

The diseases most strongly related to socioeconomic status within each country vary from one country to another. France for instance has very large inequalities in alcohol-related causes of death and in cancers, whereas for deaths from heart disease it has a slight inverse gradient. In contrast to France, both Sweden and England have much smaller inequalities in mortality from cancers, but show substantially higher rates of heart disease lower down the social scale (Kunst and Mackenbach, forthcoming 1996). There seems to be a tendency for countries having an unusually high death rate from a particular cause to have within it particularly large socioeconomic differences in death rates from the same cause. Examples include alcohol-related deaths in France, deaths from violence in the United States, and from heart disease and respiratory diseases in England and Wales. This might imply that the way of life of the upper socioeconomic groups in each country is more internationalised and so more homogeneous across countries. In contrast, lower socioeconomic groups are perhaps more likely to show the cultural characteristics particular to each country.

However, despite the differences from one country to another in the diseases which are most closely related to the extent of socioeconomic inequality within each country, we can still ask whether there are signs of any common patterns which run across a number of nations. Do some causes of death tend to be higher wherever socioeconomic or income differences are bigger?

Recent work intended to cast light on the nature of the relationship (described in chapter 5) between income distribution and life expectancy, broke down the association with life expectancy into cause-specific death rates that contribute to it (McIsaac and Wilkinson 1995). The aim was to find out if there were some causes of death which were particularly closely related to income distribution as it varied among a number of the countries with rich market economies. If so, the kind of causes of death involved might indicate something of the social processes underlying the relationship.

Despite important methodological difficulties, a fairly clear and plausible pattern did emerge. While all the major causal groupings – infections, cancers, ischaemic heart disease, other circulatory diseases, respiratory disease, chronic liver disease and accidents – tended to be more common in countries with wider income differences, some were much more affected than others. The weakest relationship among these major causal groups was that with all cancers. The strongest relationships with income distribution were found with deaths from chronic liver disease and cirrhosis, traffic accidents, infections, and – particularly among young men – deaths from injuries other than traffic accidents. These all showed a tendency to be more common in countries where income differences were larger. (This does not means that other diseases – such as heart disease – are not strongly related to income differences in at least some countries. It means only that they are not strongly related in most countries.)

If income distribution affected national standards of health primarily through the levels of chronic stress in society, then this is a group of causes of death one might reasonably expect to find implicated. Deaths from chronic liver disease and cirrhosis are likely to include a large component of alcohol- and drug-related deaths. (Unfortunately, drug-related deaths are split in the international classification between several different headings.) Throughout society alcohol is used (as we noted earlier) to help people relax, to ease social contact, to drown sorrows and escape stressful circumstances. Various other drugs which might contribute to chronic liver disease have similar uses.

Even more interesting however is the contribution of accidents. Take first death rates from road accidents, which are closely correlated with income distribution internationally. While there is a component related to alcohol consumption, accidents are also likely to be very sensitive to people's attitude to others in society at large and to public behaviour. The influence of driver behaviour on traffic accidents takes place against a background of technological improvements in the design and safety of cars and roads which have tended to bring accident rates down internationally. What the statistics suggest is that accident rates are nevertheless higher in countries with wider income differences. Perhaps nothing is so indicative of the standards of people's behaviour towards unknown others in society than aspects of the way people drive. Safety depends on drivers' courtesy to one another, on their willingness to give way at pedestrian crossings, to allow other drivers to enter traffic streams from side roads, to forgive minor errors, to obey speed limits and other traffic regulations, and to consider the safety of pedestrians – particularly children – in urban streets. The more competitive, aggressive, uncooperative, lawless, reckless and inconsiderate drivers are, the more dangerous roads get. In many ways driving behaviour is likely to be a highly sensitive reflection of how people see themselves as related to unknown members of the public in society at large. Do people see other members of the public as fellow citizens with whom their welfare is interdependent, or do they see each other merely as obstacles in each other's way?

This does not of course apply to road safety alone. Accidents other than road accidents are also related to income distribution – particularly if income distribution is measured among young single people without children who lead lives particularly prone to accidents (McIsaac and Wilkinson 1995). These will include some drug deaths and will be partly influenced by how much people value their own lives. Concern for the safety of others often means avoiding dangers which might harm the unwary. To avoid exposing others to dangers and hazards of all kinds means having regard to the welfare of unknown others and thinking of protecting them. Safe societies will be well-ordered societies, with low levels of vandalism, in which people experience themselves as part of a community with common interests.

In addition to alcohol and accidents, the tendency for death rates from infections to be higher in countries with wider income differences is also understandable in terms of the effects which stress is known to have on the immune system. Although heart disease is closely related to income differences in some countries, in general the association is weak – though stronger among women than men. Psychoneuroendocrinology provides possible explanations of why heart disease is related to socioeconomic stress.

Data available for fifty states of the United States provide one of the best statistical bases on which to analyse the effects of income distribution. As we saw in chapter 5, studies using these data show the expected pattern of higher overall mortality rates in states in which income inequalities are greatest (Kaplan, G.A. *et al.* 1996; Kennedy, B.P. *et al.* 1996). The relationship is little changed when it is controlled for the much weaker effects of average incomes or absolute poverty. But what is particularly interesting in the present context is that the association between income distribution and both the homicide rate and the rate of violent crime is even stronger than that between income distribution and total mortality. Figure 8.1 shows the correlation between homicide rates and the share of total household income received by the least well-off 50 per cent of the population across the forty-six states for which data is available. (I am indebted to Kaplan and Lynch who very generously gave me this data before publishing it themselves (see Kaplan *et al.* 1996).) Adjusting for the log of median income in each state marginally increases the strength of the correlation from the 0.72 (P<0.001) shown in figure 8.1. These correlations suggest that differences in income inequality may account for as much as half the very large differences in homicide rates from one state to another (they vary from 2 to 18 per 100,000 population per year). Earlier reports showing that homicide rates in the United States are more closely related to income inequality than to absolute poverty confirm these results (Balkwell 1990; Crutchfield 1989; Blaus and Blaus 1982; Currie 1985).

A much earlier report using data from the period 1967–73 for the 192 Standard Metropolitan Statistical Areas of the United States found clear relationships between most of the major categories of crime and the size of the 'income gap' between the incomes of the poorest 20 per cent of the population and average incomes in each area (Braithwaite 1979). National differences in the classification and reporting of crime are a serious obstacle to international comparative studies. Homicide is one of the few categories of crime which does allow cross-country comparisons to be made. Using data from thirty-one countries, Braithwaite and Braithwaite (1980) also showed a statistically significant relationship between greater inequality of earnings and higher homicide rates. Messner (1982) found that the extent of income inequality accounted for 35 per cent of the differences in homicide rates among the thirty-nine countries for which he had data.

That the links between crime and income inequality to some extent parallel those between health and inequality is highly indicative of the channels through which health is affected. It not only

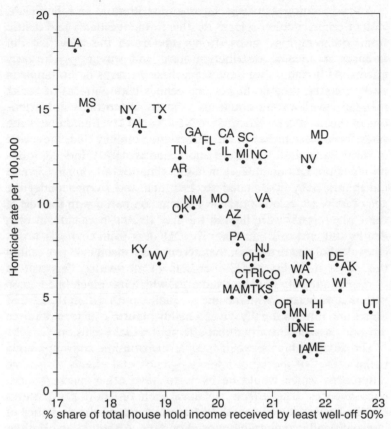

Figure 8.1: The relationship between income distribution and homicide among the states of the USA in 1990
Source: Data calculated from US Census and National Centre for Health Statistics by Kaplan, Pamuk, Lynch, Cohen and Balfour (1996) who kindly provided it for publication here

provides independent confirmation that income distribution has important psychosocial effects on society, but shows that the effects are consistent with the view that wider income differences are socially divisive. Indeed, there are suggestions that they undermine the legitimacy of the society's institutions more widely. A study which (perhaps rather too conveniently) measured political unrest in countries at different stages of development by the death rate from riots, bombings and assassinations, found that these deaths were also associated with income distribution (Pavin 1973).

An association between income distribution and homicide, violent crime, alcohol-related deaths, traffic accidents and deaths from 'other injuries' gives strong support to the view that differences in income distribution have widespread psychosocial effects. Although, as we have seen, these patterns do not apply in every country, they do find strong echoes with patterns of health inequality within some countries. A study of mortality in Harlem, one of the most deprived areas of New York City, found that death rates there were higher at most ages after infancy than they were in rural Bangladesh (McCord and Freeman 1990). Indeed, a boy born and brought up in Harlem has less chance of living to 65 years old than a baby in Bangladesh. For men and women under the age of 65 years, relative risks in Harlem compared with the rest of the United States were highest for drug deaths, homicide, alcohol deaths and cirrhosis – in that order. Deaths from cirrhosis, homicide, alcohol and drugs together accounted for some 43 per cent of the excess mortality and 30 per cent of all deaths. This pattern of raised mortality in a deprived area, which has much in common with that associated with income inequality both within the United States and internationally, gives a highly plausible picture of raised mortality associated with direct effects of social exclusion.

The relationship between income distribution and apparently social causes of mortality implies psychosocial effects of income differences which would be likely to have other marked social consequences. The effects we have seen on mortality patterns are the easiest consequences to trace because of the existence of internationally comparable mortality data. Although associations with homicide, some other kinds of crime, and with the proportion of the population imprisoned, have all been shown within the United States (Kaplan 1996, Braithwaite 1979), hard data are often lacking on other social indicators which might reflect the psychosocial effects of income distribution.

Lack of internationally comparable data may mean that it is sometimes easier to look at trends over time within a single country than to compare different countries at a point in time. Usually changes in income distribution are too small and too slow for it to be reasonable to expect to identify their effects. Indeed, economists used to regard income differentials as mysteriously stable – almost as an economic constant. However, in Britain during the 1980s income differences widened more rapidly than they had ever been recorded to have done before, and more rapidly than they had in any other developed country (with the possible exception of New Zealand) (Hills 1995). The trends were shown in figure 5.9. The point to note is that after widening slowly, income distribution started to widen very rapidly from about 1985. This provides an important opportunity to look for the psychosocial imprint of widening income differences.

As we saw in chapter 5, the widening of income differences during the later 1980s was accompanied by a slowing down in the rate of improvement in national mortality rates among age groups below 45 years old (figure 5.10), and by a widening of differences in death rates between richer and poorer areas of the country (Phillimore *et al.* 1994; McLoone and Boddy 1994; Greater Glasgow Health Board 1993). This pattern seems to have been accompanied by an almost exactly similar pattern in the results of tests of children's reading ability (Wilkinson 1994c). Because some Local Education Authorities (LEAs) in Britain have administered standard reading tests to primary school children each year, this is one of the few psychosocially sensitive outcome measures for which there is hard data. The first warning of a decline in standards came from an anonymous group of educational psychologists who claimed that reading standards had declined in the LEAs in which they worked, 'particularly during the period since 1985' (Gorman and Fernandes 1992). As well as stimulating a controversy about teaching methods, this also stimulated further research. The Schools Examinations and Assessment Council commissioned the National Foundation for Educational Research (NFER) to review the evidence on changes in reading standards of 7 year old children during the 1980s. They started with a trawl of the LEAs which had records of children's reading test results. Nineteen of the twenty-six that reported said that standards had declined and that the downward trend had 'emerged most clearly after 1985' (Gorman and Fernandes 1992). In case the impression of a decline resulted from reporting bias, they looked at results from a random sample of schools. Because of changes in reading tests, they were obliged to limit their comparison to the period 1987–91. The results confirmed that there had indeed been a decline in reading standards. Lastly, an educational psychologist in Buckinghamshire LEA, where the same reading tests had been used on all children in the Authority's schools throughout the 1980s, analysed the trends in their reading standards. The results are shown in figure 8.2 which should be compared with figures 5.9 (p. 95) and 5.10 (p. 97).

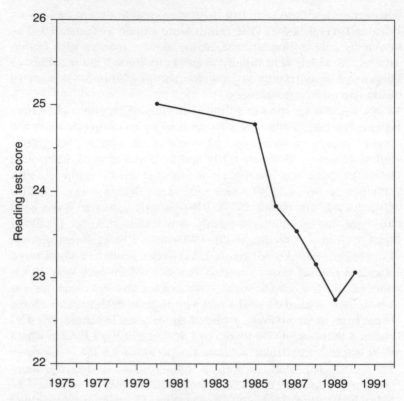

Figure 8.2: The decline in reading standards. (Chiltern reading test scores for all 7–8 year old Buckinghamshire schoolchildren)
Source: M. Lake, *Language and Learning*, June, no. 6. 1991.

Commenting on the decline, the author says '1985 is clearly a watershed year as suggested also in Turner's data' (Lake 1991). All authorities agree that there was a decline in reading standards and that it emerged particularly clearly from 1985.

From the beginning, Conservative Ministers of Education had blamed the decline in reading standards on the so-called 'real books' method of teaching reading, but researchers found no significant associations between the teaching method and children's reading performance. Indeed, only a small minority of schools used the real books method and, if anything, their numbers declined during the period. The lack of an association with methods of teaching reading was confirmed by a report from Croydon Education Authority which said that there had been a parallel decline in children's performance in mathematics (London Borough of Croydon 1992). The only correlates of the decline in standards were the socioeconomic characteristics of the area. The NFER reported that half the schools in which standards had fallen were in large conurbations and industrial centres, while none of the schools which showed a rise in performance were inner city schools or in areas of deprivation (Gorman and Fernandes 1992). Rather than an all-round decline in reading standards, there was apparently an increase in the proportion of children in the lowest scoring group. In Buckinghamshire the pattern was for a decline in standards among the schools in the poorest neighbourhoods, which was more than enough to offset the small improvements which took place in schools in better areas. This is exactly the pattern we saw behind the trends in mortality. Confirming that the effect was unrelated to the schools themselves, one of the psychological tests used suggested that the problem was associated with a deterioration in the quality of the home background of the less able readers (Lake 1991).

There can be little doubt that children's reading abilities were affected by rising material inequalities in much the same way as the death rates of infants, of children and of people in the parental age range (figure 5.10, p. 97). The socioeconomic pattern and the timing of the trends are almost identical.

Between 1979 and 1991 there was a threefold increase in the proportion of children living in families on incomes below half the national average – which is the European Union's relative income poverty line (Department of Social Security 1993). With almost a third of the nation's children coming from homes in relative poverty, it is likely that in poorer areas as many as a half or two-thirds of the children in every classroom would come from families facing the problems of poverty. Inevitably teaching and learning become more difficult in such conditions. Classrooms would have more disruptive children and more children with behavioural problems and emotional disturbances. Pointing in the same direction is the increase in school expulsions which the Advisory Centre for Education (ACE) documented over the years 1986–91 (Advisory Centre for Education 1993). During these years there was a rapid growth in expulsions from both primary and secondary schools. Although it seemed likely that schools may have changed their attitude to 'difficult' children and expelled more of them as a result of the introduction of the 'local management of schools' policy, ACE reported that there was no statistical relationship between the rate at which LEAs delegated their powers to schools in different areas and the rate at which expulsions increased.

Several reports suggest, on the basis of fairly poor evidence, that there has been an increase in the proportion of children with behavioural disturbances. Certainly 40 of 52 LEAs which answered an inquiry believed that the frequency of behavioural problems in their schools had increased (Bennathan and Smith 1991). Only one thought otherwise.

There are a number of other trends suggestive of the effects of widening income differences in Britain during the later 1980s. From 1987 violent crime in England and Wales rose at an unprecedented rate – faster than at any time since the Second World War. In a thorough survey of the research, James (1995) shows how this is partly a lagged effect of the stress experienced by the rapidly growing number of families with children living in relative poverty, and partly the more immediate effects of relative poverty. Relative poverty increased more rapidly in the early 1980s among families with children than it did among other sections of society. James shows that violent young men were often violent as children and that the most important risk factors are parental irritability and disharmony, as well as depression and violence consequent on relative poverty. He provides very convincing evidence that the extraordinarily rapid rise in 'violence against the person' was directly attributable to widening income differentials.

Although suicide rates are often inversely associated with violence against others, in Britain suicide rates among young men 15–24 years old rose by 75 per cent during the mid and later 1980s (OPCS 1991). The rise has been shown to be related to growing socioeconomic inequalities. Indeed, the rise in suicide was the main component of the rising mortality rates among young men and women (20–29 years) in the poorest Scottish postcode areas between 1981 and 1991 (McLoone and Boddy 1994). As relative deprivation in these areas increased, the 'all causes' mortality rates of young men rose by 29 per cent and young women by 11 per cent. The rise in suicide is likely to have been particularly closely related to rising unemployment (Platt and Kreitman 1984).

However, internationally suicide does not appear to be more common in countries where income differences are wider – indeed there are signs that the reverse is true (McIsaac and Wilkinson 1996). The international picture is likely to reflect the inverse relationship between suicide and homicide rates which has been observed both before and since Durkheim's famous study of suicide (Ferri 1895; Durkheim 1952; James 1995). The implication is that whether the anger and bitterness goes inwards or outwards, whether you blame others or yourself, is affected by the social context. Despite the association between suicide and unemployment in Britain, the picture in parts of the United States is different. Of the seventeen causes of death shown in the study of mortality in Harlem, suicide was the only cause for which rates were actually lower in Harlem than among whites in the US as a whole (McCord and Freeman 1990).

Between the early 1980s and 1991 there was more than a doubling of drug dealing offences recorded by the police in Britain. Drug offences among young people increased particularly rapidly (Joseph Rowntree Foundation 1993). The fourfold or fivefold increase in deaths from sniffing glue and other volatile substances suggests that the change was not merely a change in reporting (Taylor *et al.* 1993). The Institute for the Study of Drug Dependence reported: 'The relatively stable youth drug use patterns of the mid 1980s were disturbed in the late 1980s, and by the 1990s there was increased use of established drugs like cannabis, solvents, amphetamines, and magic mushrooms and an upsurge in the use of ecstasy and LSD.' The links between increased relative poverty, drug use and crime during this period have also been traced in a local study of the Wirral in Liverpool (Parker *et al.* 1988).

One of the ways in which adverse socioeconomic circumstances may do lasting psychological and emotional damage is through increasing the level of stress in which domestic life is lived. The social and economic environment establishes many of the difficulties with which domestic life has to cope and cannot be separated from a range of what are normally seen as family problems. It is not just that worries about money, jobs and housing spill over into domestic conflict as tempers become more quickly frayed and parents find themselves with smaller reserves of patience and tolerance. It is also that lack of money, of choices, play space, the need for enough indoor space to accommodate incompatible family activities – in short, the lack of resources of all kinds (including time) – means that people's needs and demands are brought into conflict with each other. The tighter the constraints within which a family must operate, the fewer the demands which can be satisfied, and the more people's interests conflict. The smaller the resources, the less the capacity to overcome unforeseen difficulties, accidents, breakages or losses. The greater the potential sources of stress and conflict, the more family life and social support will suffer. For example, a study of the effects of unemployment on marriage found that half the couples reported an increase in the number of arguments and a third said that one or other partner had left home temporarily or contemplated doing so (Burgoyne 1985). Social life was curtailed and their circle of friends shrank. Other studies have shown – predictably – that deprivation causes stress, that socioeconomic status affects 'fatalism and attributional style' (Wheaton 1980), that economic hardship reduces people's ability to fulfil their roles – whether as 'breadwinner' or 'homemaker' – and so causes depression (Ross and Huber 1985). A Swedish study found that family dissension in childhood was associated with more than a 50 per cent increase in mortality among men and women aged 30–75 (Lundberg 1993).

In fact, this last study reported that death rates in adulthood among people who had experienced family dissension during their childhood were higher than among those who had experienced economic hardship in childhood. Similarly, in a cohort of 17,000 people followed up since birth in 1958, Power found that the best predictor of their health when they were 23 years old was an assessment of their behaviour made by teachers when they were 16 years old. Those identified by teachers using the Rutter Behaviour Scale as showing 'deviant' behaviour – 'emotional or conduct disorders' – scored much less well on health measures when aged 23, even after taking other social and economic factors into account (Power *et al.* 1991). Findings like these on the relative importance of material and psychosocial factors may reflect problems of measurement, but they are likely to indicate that the effects of economic factors are transmitted largely through psychosocial channels. Given that economic factors increase the risks of psychosocial difficulties – but are far from being their only cause – it is perfectly possible that the links between psychosocial factors and health might be stronger than those between material factors and health. Indeed, that this is so suggests that psychosocial factors provide the primary links between material disadvantage and health.

Even without these examples showing that a range of problems worsens as income differences widen, the strength of the association between relative material deprivation and a number of social problems is familiar to everyone. We all know that as well as worse health, poor areas have more than their share of crime, low educational performance, drug abuse and violence. The correlation between, for example, the Department of the Environment's deprivation scores for local education authorities and GCSE exam results for 16 year olds is 0.81, suggesting that two-thirds of the variation in results between areas is a reflection of differences in deprivation. (The correlation between the same deprivation score and mortality was 0.76 for men and 0.58 for women (Morris *et al.* 1996). Another deprivation index – the Townsend Index – shows higher correlations with mortality (Phillimore *et al.* 1994).)

How these area-based measures are related to domestic circumstances, family stress and to the lives of individual children, is not hard to imagine. If we take child abuse as the partly visible tip of the much more widespread problem of domestic conflict, it is notable that the top three contributory sources of stress which caseworkers write down when registering each case of child abuse are: marital problems, debts and unemployment (Creighton 1992). The scale of the wider problem is clearly illustrated in findings from a study of 15,000 children aged 10 years born in 1970 (see figure 10.2, p. 206). Rates of hyperactivity were over three times as high, and conduct disorders four times as high, in social class V (unskilled manual occupations) as in social class I (professional occupations) (Woodroffe *et al.* 1993).

The family's external environment, the circumstances into which domestic life has to fit, has a dramatic impact on the chances either of maintaining stable, caring relationships or – alternatively – of disintegration into conflict and violence. Anything which increases the tensions and difficulties of family life will decrease tolerance and increase conflict, thereby adding to the numbers of children with behavioural problems and learning difficulties, and to those who at older ages are more likely to be unemployed and to be involved with drugs and crime. Domestic conflict is extraordinarily damaging to children's emotional welfare and substantially outweighs the effects of being brought up by one rather than two parents. Although children of divorced or separated parents (as opposed to parents who have always brought up children on their own) do show significant developmental disadvantages, the indication – from studies which have followed up large numbers of children – is that these disadvantages usually start before couples separate and reflect the emotional impact of the parental conflict which led to the divorce or separation (Wadsworth *et al.* 1990; Ferri and Robinson 1976). If developmental measures taken of children after their parents got divorced are controlled by measures taken before the divorce (which effectively controls for the signs of damage which preceded the divorce), there is very little sign of additional damage which can be attributed to being brought up by only one parent. Family process is much more important than family structure (Sweeting and West 1995).

In terms of the policy implications it is very important to distinguish the effects of having one parent from the effects of living in greater poverty as most of the children of single parents do. In Britain in 1990/1, 74 per cent of children in single-parent families lived on less than half the average income (household income adjusted to take account of the number of people in each household) (Department of Social Security 1993). This rise, from 28 per cent in 1979, represents more than a two-and-a-half-fold increase in the proportion of all children of single parents who live in relative poverty. Rather than seeing the profound social effects of widening income differences and increasing relative poverty, a growing range of social problems are laid at the door of single-parent families. However, when you compare children of lone parents with equally poor children brought up by both parents, most of the differences disappear (McLanahan 1985; Ferri 1976). Similarly, children of the small proportion of better-off lone parents do as well as children in better-off two-parent families: almost all the educational and developmental disadvantage seems to be explained by the degree of poverty.

In the context of the frequent arguments about the effects of being brought up in lone parent families, the similarities and differences between Sweden and Japan are illuminating. They show very clearly that much the most important problem is not family structure but relative poverty. In terms of family structure, they are at opposite ends of the spectrum. Among developed market economies, Japan clings closest to the traditional two-parent nuclear family, with few divorces and few births outside marriage. In contrast, more than half of all births in Sweden are outside marriage – a total exceeded only by Iceland. However, despite the enormous difference between them, they both have the highest standards of child health and welfare. In terms of the death rates among children under 5 years old (the most important international indicator of child welfare used by UNICEF), Sweden has the lowest rate in the world and Japan comes second (UNICEF 1993). What both countries also had in common was a much more egalitarian distribution of income: again, among the developed market economies, Japan had the narrowest income differences with Sweden close behind. Figures from 1987 show that in Sweden only 2 per cent of lone parent families lived in relative poverty (below half the average income) compared with an average of 21.2 per cent among a group of OECD countries (Hewlett 1993). In the United States some 54 per cent of the children of lone parents were living in relative poverty (Hewlett 1993), a proportion which official figures suggests was close to that for the United Kingdom when these comparisons were made (Department of Social Security 1993). This is no doubt part of the explanation of why infant mortality rates among babies born to single parents in Sweden were lower even than the rates for babies born within marriage in social class I professional families in Britain (see figure 5.7) (Leon *et al.* 1992). The difference between countries in which children do well and those in which they do badly is therefore not family structure but the extent of relative poverty among their families and the stresses this imposes on family life.

Another important feature of Japan in the present context is that it is probably the only developed country to have had substantial long-term reductions in crime. The only category of crime which has not decreased is what is referred to in the Japanese statistics as 'intellectual crimes' – which actually means fraud and white-collar crime (Statistics Bureau, Japan 1990). Reflecting the influence on the crime rate of progressively narrowing income differences during the postwar decades, crime has decreased most in the inner city areas where it was highest, and its association with social class and poverty has progressively weakened (Clifford 1976). The categories of crime which have decreased, namely homicide, robbery, rape, violence and bodily injury, include those which have been shown – in international studies as well as within the United States – to be associated with income distribution. Sweden is sometimes cited as a country where narrower income differences are not associated with lower crime rates. However, figures from the International Crime Survey show it is not a counter-example.

That crime as well as health and welfare are associated with income distribution provides important additional evidence as to the mechanisms involved. Although we have talked loosely of 'socioeconomic stress', what we need to know is how social processes related to social inequality and division have their greatest psychological purchase on us. It is clear that there are important links through domestic stress. These are particularly important in young children on whom they are likely to have life-long effects. (We shall look briefly at evidence on that in chapter 10.) During adult life it is not clear whether, at the physiological level, there are distinct forms of stress, or whether there is only one form of generalised chronic stress. Epidemiologists have identified a number of the sources of stress which affect health in adult life which we shall discuss in the next chapter. These include lack of a sense of control over one's situation, lack of social support, poor social networks, depression and low self-esteem. Research on crime raises some important additional possibilities.

In a study of homicide, Daly and Wilson (1988) suggest that 'loss of face' is the most common source of violence. Loss of face boils down to a loss of pride, humiliation or loss of prestige in the eyes of others. Although the focus of attention here is the nature of the particular situations with which an individual might be confronted, it is not hard to imagine that people with larger reserves of status and prestige may feel less fundamentally threatened by any particular loss of face. More interesting, however, is the argument which Braithwaite develops in his *Crime, shame and reintegration* (1989). His theory of 'reintegrative shaming' is essentially a theory of socialisation which is as relevant to child rearing as to crime control. Drawing on child development research, he says that effective socialisation depends on being able to discipline children within the context of continuing love and care, which the child knows will continue beyond any punishment or expression of disapproval. 'Families in which disapproval rather than approval is the normal state of affairs are incapable of socializing children by with-drawal of approval' (Braithwaite 1989, p. 56). The effectiveness of withdrawal of approval depends on the contrast with the normal enjoyment of approval. This must be the fundamental basis of socialisation in all societies, and Braithwaite argues that the same processes are the basis of social control throughout adult life. Citing a great deal of research, he says that although there is an association between lower offending and a greater likelihood of being caught, there is little evidence of an association between crime rates and the severity of punishment. He concludes: 'It would seem that sanctions imposed by relatives, friends or a personally relevant collectivity have more effect on criminal behaviour than sanctions imposed by a remote legal authority' (ibid., p. 69). Repute in the eyes of close acquaintances appears to matter more to people than the opinions or actions of criminal justice officials. Of young men asked what would be the most important consequence of being arrested, a large majority said it would be what their families and girlfriends thought about it and the shame and publicity of appearing in court. Less than one-sixth as many said it would be the kind of punishment they received. Braithwaite sees the existence of a moral community, and of maintaining people within it, as fundamental. Shaming can be destructive if it is stigmatising instead of reintegrative because it pushes people out of the moral community into dissident subcultures. He also illustrates the power of social or moral motivation by quoting an experiment in which people were interviewed within a month of having to fill out tax returns. To one group the interviewer stressed the strict penalties for income tax evasion, while to the other the moral reasons for tax compliance were emphasised. The moral appeal led to a significantly greater increase in the amount of tax paid (Schwartz and Orleans 1967).

After pointing out that although 45 per cent of those convicted of a crime serve jail sentences in the USA compared to less than 2 per cent in Japan, Braithwaite uses Bayley's study of Japanese and American policing to illustrate how integrative shaming can work in a modern developed society.

> [Japanese] offenders against the law are expected to accept the community's terms for resocialization rather than insisting on legal innocence and bargaining for mitigation of punishment. . . . Individual character is thought mutable [and] responsive to informal sanctions of proximate groups; . . . individuals feel a moral obligation to assist actively in preserving the moral consensus in the community.
>
> (Bayley 1976, p. 196)

> Japanese policemen seek more than compliance, they seek acceptance of the community's moral values. They are not merely the law's enforcers; they are teachers in the virtue of the law. The Japanese police have been given a moral mandate, based on recognition of their importance in shaping the polity.
>
> (ibid., p. 186)

Some of Bayley's descriptions sound unlikely to Western ears:

In psychological terms, the system relies on positive rather than negative reinforcement, emphasizing loving acceptance in exchange for genuine repentance. An analogue of what the Japanese policeman wants the offender to feel is the tearful relief of a child when confession of wrongdoing to his parents results in a gentle laugh and a warm hug. In relation to an American policeman, Japanese officers want to be known for the warmth of their care rather than the strictness of their enforcement.

(ibid., p. 156)

These remarkable descriptions of Japanese policing are probably less important for the direct influence they may have on crime than they are as an indication of the highly integrated nature of Japanese society within which crime rates are determined.

On the effects of low social integration, Durkheim said 'The more weakened the groups to which [a person] belongs, the less he depends on them, the more he consequently depends only on himself and recognises no other rules of conduct than what are founded in his private interests' (Durkheim 1952, p. 209). Conversely, in a cohesive society there is 'a constant interchange of ideas and feelings from all to each and each to all, something like a mutual moral support, which instead of throwing the individual on his own resources, leads him to share in the collective energy and supports his own when exhausted' (ibid., p. 210).

Durkheim's work on social integration was part of his analysis of the social causes of suicide. He believed that high suicide rates could arise from any of three dimensions of the relationship between the individual and the moral community. One was altruistic suicide, in which the social control of the individual was so strong that people may feel obliged to kill themselves as a matter of honour or duty. At the opposite pole was egotistical suicide, in which the social integration and collective activity is too weak to sustain people in the wider social purposes and processes of society. The third was anomic suicide, which again comes from 'society's insufficient presence in the individual' (ibid., p. 258), without which – he believed – people were more likely to have unrealistic goals and to become detached from the structure of attainable norms and limitations which they could handle.

It is clear that poorer health and higher rates of crime, particularly violent crime, are strongly associated with the weaker social integration which Durkheim associated with egotistical suicide. Although some suicide has an egotistic or anomic pattern – as can be seen from its association with unemployment (Platt and Kreitman 1984), suicide and homicide are usually inversely related (Ferri 1895; James 1995). The fact that suicides are now rather more common in societies with narrower income differences (McIsaac and Wilkinson 1996) suggests that higher rates of suicide occur in more highly integrated societies, perhaps because of a sense of shame when people feel they have let down their family, colleagues or community.

Durkheim drew attention to some of the most important ways in which societies differ. However, the unrelenting processes of social differentiation which reflect and amplify social hierarchy are fundamentally important in any analysis of social integration and community. It is these processes which create social exclusion, which stigmatise the most deprived and establish social distances throughout society. These processes are fed and nurtured by inequalities of what Bourdieu calls economic and cultural capital. Bourdieu has shown how differences in taste – in almost every sphere of life – are not only closely associated with differences in income and wealth, in education and in individual social capital, but are used to express these social distinctions in terms of superiority and inferiority (Bourdieu 1984). As he says, 'Sociology is rarely more akin to social psychoanalysis than when it confronts an object like taste, one of the most vital stakes in the struggles fought in the field of the dominant class and the field of cultural production' (ibid., p. 11). The methods he describes for creating and expressing social distinction are presumably closely related to the sense of inferiority which Sennett and Cobb picked out as a key component of American manual workers' experience of class in their study *The hidden injuries of class* (1971).

In terms of the basis for processes of social stratification and social distinction, we can probably regard income distribution as a proxy for inequalities in both economic and educational capital. Because processes of social differentiation feed on these inequalities and destroy social cohesion, the extent to which we have an integrated and harmonious society with high levels of social involvement, or at the other extreme a society that is divided, dominated by status, prejudice and social exclusion, which gives rise to aggressive subgroups antagonistic to the rest of society, and the stigmatisation of the most disadvantaged, will be closely related to the extent of income inequality. As people in early forms of society recognised only too well, you cannot achieve social integration without economic integration. The values of social life will tend to reflect the principles of economic life.

Part IV

How society kills

Chapter 9

The psychosocial causes of illness

It is not yet possible to identify with any precision the main pathways that link the social cohesion of the egalitarian societies discussed in chapter 6 to the higher standards of physical health and longevity which their populations enjoy. Rather than thinking of psychosocial influences on health as weak, disputed and entirely secondary to more powerful material influences on health, the evidence seems to warrant the opposite view – at least of the determinants of health in the developed countries. We saw in chapter 3 that health in rich societies that have gone through the epidemiological transition is no longer limited primarily by the direct effects of material factors. Having attained basic minimum standards for the vast majority of the population, it looks increasingly as if the psychosocial influences on health are pre-eminent.

We no longer have to evoke images of voodoo death to argue that psychosocial stress can kill. Fortunately there is now a great deal of epidemiological and experimental evidence which removes any doubt that psychosocial factors can exert very powerful influences on physical health – both morbidity and mortality. This chapter starts off with a brief sketch of the evidence, which shows the enormous range of possibilities for such links. The problem is not so much that there is a shortage of potential pathways, but that there are a vast number of possibilities which are all quite plausible in the light of what is already known. The work which is needed to rule out some and confirm the importance of others will take some years.

Relative income is an inherently social concept. It reflects an aspect of the relationship of an individual to a social group. Because we are trying to explain the health effects of low relative rather than absolute income, we will concentrate on psychological and social pathways. The importance of income distribution implies that we must explain the effect of low income on health through its social meanings and implications for social position rather than through the direct physical effects which material circumstances might have independently of their social connotations in any particular society. This is not to say that bad (or even non-existent) housing and an inadequate diet do not affect the health of a minority (though still a large number) of people in developed societies: they clearly do. What it means is that the direct material effects of factors such as these are not the main explanations of why national standards of health are related to income distribution. Nor does this mean that we shall ignore the health of the poorest in society. The poor suffer the psychosocial effects of deprivation as well as its direct material effects. Indeed, it is important to recognise that as well as the greatest material deprivation, those at the bottom of the social hierarchy also suffer the greatest social, psychological and emotional deprivation, and this may well have a greater impact on their health than the more direct effects of material deprivation.

Even among those living in what must by any standards have been absolute material poverty, Sapolsky has provided remarkable evidence of the physiological marks of the unremitting nature of the socioeconomic stress they lived with (Sapolsky 1991). After describing how almost all of the dead bodies used to teach anatomy in London medical schools in the century 1830–1930 came from poorhouses, Sapolsky says that the adrenal gland was thought to be much larger than is now regarded as normal. When anatomists saw the occasional adrenal gland from someone richer, they noted it was oddly smaller and invented a new disease – *idiopathic adrenal atrophy* – to explain it. This 'disease' flourished in the early twentieth century until physicians realised that the smaller adrenal glands were the norm and the disorder was transformed into an 'embarrassing footnote' in medical texts. The enlarged adrenals of the poor were the result of prolonged socioeconomic stress. Similarly, the thymus gland, essential to the immune system, was often shrunken away among the poor who had become accustomed to chronic stress. The larger thymus glands found in the bodies of the better-off were once again seen as a disorder and, Sapolsky says, treated with radiation which later caused thyroid cancer.

Hence, even in historical periods when the main problem was absolute rather than relative poverty for a much larger proportion of the population, the physical impact of the extreme psycho-social and emotional stress which came with it should not be underestimated. The material insecurity is itself a source of stress: it is a constant threat and source of worry which often gives way to despair. Pictures such as Hogarth's *Gin Lane* leave no room to doubt that poverty affects health most powerfully through psycho-social channels – even among the poor in eighteenth-century London.

An indication of the importance of stress in the context of depri-vation in modern society comes from a prisoner writing of life in the 1990s in an English prison (probably still not the worst in the developed world). He said: 'The end of the day leaves the nerves so taut that you jerk and jive as you unwind towards sleep. The first rattle of keys in the morning brings fear' (Shannon and Morgan 1996).

Another approach to thinking about the comparative impor-tance of psychosocial and direct material pathways in the link between income and health, is to consider housing. Although people in bad housing have much higher rates of the main cancers and heart disease, almost no one suggests that physical aspects of bad housing make an important direct contribution to these causes of death (Lowry 1991). However, there is evidence that damp housing contributes directly to the excess of respiratory disease via the increase of mould spores in the air. But first, such respiratory illnesses are a very small part of the burden of increased ill-health associated with bad housing; and second, surveys of housing conditions suggest that perhaps as little as 7 per cent of the total population live in damp housing (Ineichen 1993). Even if this is a gross underestimate, it is clear that we need to think primarily about the social implications of relative deprivation when trying to understand not only the association between health and poor housing, but more particularly when trying to explain the relation-ship between income distribution and the health of the population as a whole.

One of the clearest indications that relative deprivation affects health through psychosocial channels has come from studies of the health effects of unemployment. One of the initial difficulties facing research in this field was the possible scale of selection: were the unemployed less healthy because unemployment really damages health, or was it just that unhealthy people were more likely to become unemployed? Simple comparisons of the health of the employed and the unemployed could not distinguish between these two possibilities. Only when evidence from factory closures studies – causing unselective unemployment – became available, was it shown conclusively that health really did deteriorate *as a consequence* of unemployment. But, even more interesting, these same studies also showed that much of the deterioration in health started, not when people actually became unemployed, but before that – when redundancies were first announced. It now turns out that a large part of the link between health and unemployment is related to job insecurity and the anticipation of unemployment. This has now been demonstrated at least four times (Iversen and Klausen 1981; Ferrie *et al.* 1995; Cobb and Kasl 1977; Mattiasson *et al.* 1990). It provides powerful evidence that one of the clearest categories of deprivation in modern societies affects health predominantly through psychosocial channels.

These results are also interesting because the problem of job insecurity is much more widespread than unemployment itself. While its extent will tend to vary with changes in unemployment, the growth of the 'marginal' or 'flexible' labour force will act as a powerful multiplier of job insecurity. A MORI survey found that even among the 'middle classes' (A, B, C1) in work, 35 per cent were worried about the prospects of losing their jobs within 12 months while 20 per cent of families had recent experience of unemployment (Smith 1994).

Job insecurity is presumably only one among several other categories of financial or material insecurity. A study that indicates the health effects of housing insecurity showed that the number of tenants attending their general practitioner changed according to whether the council threat to demolish their housing estate was currently 'on' or 'off'. Housing insecurity, whether caused by council plans or difficulty in keeping up with rent or mortgage payments, has much in common with fears of unemployment. The high rate of housing repossessions reflects only the tip of an iceberg of housing insecurity, yet over 75,000 homes were repossessed by building societies in Britain in 1991, and there were another 275,000 homes at least 6 months in arrears on mortgage payments (*Building Societies Yearbook* 1993/4). These figures only include owner occupiers; they say nothing about the problems of people in the rented housing sector.

The numbers of people who lose their homes are in turn only the tip of the vast numbers who live with worrying debts. So far the effects of debt on health have not been adequately researched: there are only a few papers which mention the contribution of debt and financial insecurity to the health effects of unemployment (Bartley 1994; White 1991; Wilson and Walker 1993). However, as press reports of up to thirty suicides among 'financially embarrassed' Lloyd's 'names' suggest, the health effects of debt are not confined to the poor (McGowan 1994).

Additional evidence that the nature of the link between low relative income and health is cognitive rather than simply material comes from studies in Australia and Ireland which both found that the subjective experience of 'financial stress' was more closely related to health than was the actual level of income (Ullah 1990; Whelan 1991).

While there have been studies such as these linking sources of specifically socioeconomic stress with health, there have also been more tightly controlled experiments demonstrating the underlying link between physical health and stress from a variety of sources. In one example volunteers completed a standard psychological questionnaire designed to measure their stress levels and were then randomly allocated between two groups (Cohen et al. 1991). In this blind randomised control trial, people in one group were given nasal drops of distilled water containing five varieties of cold virus; those in the control group were given nasal drops containing only pure distilled water. The results showed that there was a gradient in the proportion who developed colds which rose from 27 per cent among low-stress people to 47 per cent among those with high levels of stress. This suggests that high levels of stress may increase the chances of catching a cold by 75 per cent. The association remained even after controlling for age, sex, education, allergic status, weight and season. Nor were the differences accounted for by possible 'stress-illness mediators' such as smoking, alcohol consumption, exercise, diet or sleep loss.

Despite controlling for factors such as these, it might be argued that high- and low-stress people differed from one another in some other way which accounted for the differences in infection rates. However, a number of studies show signs of weakened immunity and poorer health associated with a clearly identifiable environmental source of stress. For example, a study which examined throat swabs from medical students during exams found that comparisons of swabs showed that exam stress weakened their immunity (Kennedy, S. et al. 1988). There is also evidence that the stress of marital breakdown and dysfunction can affect the immune system. The effects were found to be stronger the more recent the marital breakdown and the greater the attachment to the ex-partner (Kennedy, S. *et al.* 1988). A study in south Wales found that close relatives of the children killed when a slag heap from the Aberfan coal mine collapsed on a primary school had death rates seven times as high as controls during the following year (Conduit 1992). Similarly, people whose houses were flooded in Bristol had a 50 per cent increase in mortality in the following year compared to those whose homes had not been flooded (Bennet 1970).

Even conditions such as childhood accidents, in which psychological influences might seem less plausible, have been found to be strongly influenced by maternal depression. Brown concluded from his follow-up study of mothers that 'Psychiatric difficulties in the mother appear to account for much of the class differences in childhood accidents' (Brown 1978). (This is a particularly important finding given that the class gradient in childhood accidents is particularly steep.) He found that accidents among children in social class V (unskilled manual workers and their families) doubled if mothers were depressed. Rates of depression were four times as high (28 per cent) among working-class as middle-class mothers. Because the study followed mothers over a period, it was able to show that accident rates were only higher while mothers were actually depressed. In the weeks before and afterwards, their children had similar accident rates to those of women who did not suffer depression.

It has also been possible to identify increased mortality among the general population associated with a broader list of stressful 'life events'. One study which followed a cohort of 752 middle-aged men for seven years found that death rates were over three and a half times as high among those who had experienced at least three stressful life events (Rosengren 1993). In descending order of importance, their list of ten life events ran: being legally prosecuted, forced to move house, divorce or separation, serious financial trouble, feelings of insecurity at work, serious concern about a family member, serious illness in family, being made redundant, being forced to change job, and lastly, death of a family member. Even though death of a family member came last in this list, studies of bereavement have shown that the death of one partner in a marriage is likely to hasten the death of the other

(Helsing and Szklo 1981). Deaths from cancers, heart disease and alcohol-related causes were particularly high. A prospective study of people who had had a heart attack also showcd that rates of recurrence were much higher among people with long-term difficulties (Tennant *et al.* 1994).

Progress has also been made in identifying psychosocial characteristics of work which affect health. For most workers in the developed world, certainly for all office workers, the social organisation of work is now likely to be the most important occupational health hazard. Research trying to explain socioeconomic status differences in health in relation to the working environment has also come up with results which indicate the importance of psychosocial processes. Karasek and Theorell (1990) drew attention to the deleterious health effects of having little control over one's work, low social support from managers or colleagues in the workplace, and a fast pace of work. The three were independently related to cardiovascular symptoms and a number of other health problems. Marmot *et al.* (1991) have found similar relationships contributing to the threefold differences in mortality in the Whitehall study. Although the seniority of the level of employment within the Civil Service is closely related to the amount of control people have over their work, control over work was significantly related to health, even after controlling for employment grade and a number of other risk factors. Conflicting job demands and, in the absence of control, a heavy workload, were also associated with poorer health in this study.

One of the advantages of workplace studies such as these is that they can show the links all the way from the objective conditions in which people work, through to the psychosocial impact on individuals and their health. The effects of feeling in control or of personal efficacy on the one hand, and of learned helplessness on the other, have received a great deal of attention in social psychology and have been found to be important in numerous areas of performance as well as in tolerance of pain and several health outcomes. Although in much of this work these characteristics are subject to environmental manipulation – as the term 'learned helplessness' suggests – they are nevertheless often regarded as if they were fixed personality characteristics. When trying to explain the effects of socioeconomic circumstances on health, psychosocial factors are relevant only to the extent to which they are responses to those circumstances.

The importance to health of the amount of control people have over their work, the pressure of work, and the social support they get at work has now been confirmed in workplace studies in Sweden, the United States, Germany and Britain (Johnson and Hall 1988; Karasek *et al.* 1988; Siegrist *et al.* 1990; Karasek and Theorell 1990; Marmot *et al.* 1991). However, these findings are doubly significant: although studied in the working environment, they all have their domestic equivalents and are likely to tell us as much about the kinds of factors that influence health at home as they do about those at work. In many ways money is a key to the ability to control one's life. The more money, the greater one's options, the more choice and the more easily most problems can be overcome. Indeed, problems of job or housing insecurity may be seen as instances of a more general category of financial insecurity where important areas of control are lost. The importance of social support also transfers to the world outside work.

A number of studies have shown the beneficial health effects of more, and better quality, social contact between people at home or in the community (House *et al.* 1988; Broadhead *et al.* 1983; Berkman and Syme 1979). Various forms of social support and social contact are now generally accepted as having an important beneficial effect on health. It seems likely that social support may be important in changing the way people respond to stressful events and circumstances (Whelan 1993; Rosengren *et al.* 1993). Lack of a confiding relationship with a close friend, relative or partner is associated with poorer health, but so also is less involvement with wider social networks, community activities, etc.

In terms of the relationships between health and income distribution (chapter 5) and between income distribution and social cohesion (chapter 6), the evidence of the health effects of lower social involvement in the community and of less good social networks is particularly interesting. In a review, Berkman says:

> Between 1979 . . . and 1994 there have been eight community-based prospective studies that reveal an association between what we have now come to call social integration and mortality rates, usually death from all causes . . . Overall, they consistently show that people who are isolated are at increased mortality risk from a number of causes. Furthermore, they have several important methodological strengths which give us confidence in their findings. . . .

In the first of these studies, from Alameda County, men and women who lacked ties to others (in this case, based on an index assessing contacts with friends and relatives, marital status, and church and group membership) were 1.9 to 3.1 times more likely to die in a 9-year follow-up period . . . than those who had many more contacts.

(Berkman 1995, p. 246)

Berkman emphasises that the effects of a lack of social contact extend to a wide range of causes of death and influence both the incidence of disease and case-fatality rates. Indeed, she cites evidence of threefold differences in case-fatality rates after a heart attack according to whether or not patients had good social support. Several possible causal pathways linking the effects of social relations to health have been identified involving both the immune and the neuroendocrine systems.

Although the apparent importance of social relations to health provides a pleasingly direct link between social cohesion and health, there is just a possibility that the results could be explained in terms of individual selection. If more sociable people turned out to be healthier because they have different psychological characteristics, a more sociable society might not improve health through this route. Putting the usual worries about the ecological fallacy into reverse, it might be wrong to infer from individual studies to social policy for whole communities.

However, there is evidence that psychosocial interventions in other areas make a difference to health. We have seen evidence of the importance of psychosocial influences on physical health from observational studies and experiments such as the one showing a relationship between stress levels and vulnerability to experimental exposure to cold viruses. But there are also studies of the effects of interventions designed to lower stress levels by teaching people relaxation and meditation techniques. In one particularly impressive example, people with raised blood pressure were randomised between two groups, one of which was given advice on smoking, diet and exercise, while the other was also given a one-hour relaxation and stress-management class once a week for eight weeks (Patel and Marmot 1987). After eight months, and then again four years later, it was found that blood pressure was significantly lower among people in the group who were given relaxation lessons. When asked, members of this group said that although few continued to practise relaxation regularly, a number did still tell themselves to relax or calm down when dealing with stressful problems. In the present context, the importance of this – and other similar experimental interventions – is that although it would be unethical to conduct experiments which seriously increased levels of chronic stress, by lowering stress they provide almost conclusive evidence of the importance of psychosocial processes to health and indicate the possible benefits of intervention.

Many of the most important sources of stress in our lives are likely to come from the socioeconomic environment and will be exacerbated by relatively low incomes. To talk about socio-economic disadvantage affecting health through psychosocial pathways is not to suggest that the problems are in some way 'psychological' rather than 'real'. People worry about losing homes if they are unable to keep up mortgage payments or rent because that is a real danger. To emphasise psychological pathways does not mean that the basic cause of the problem is psychological or can be dealt with by psychological interventions. The point of distin-guishing psychosocial pathways from exclusively material ones is to distinguish the social and economic problems affecting health through various forms of worry, stress, insecurity, etc., and those that – like air or water pollution – affect health through wholly material pathways, even if we are totally unaware and unconcerned by them. We could talk simply of cognitive rather than psycho-social pathways, but the cognitions that are sufficiently stressful to matter are of course the ones that are particularly emotionally charged and that arise from enduring aspects of one's life circum-stances. While it would be perverse not to be worried about the prospect of losing your home if you were unable to continue paying for it, it has to be recognised how destructive such threats can be, even if the house is eventually not lost. A sense of desperation, anger, bitterness, learned helplessness or aggression are all wholly understandable responses to various social, economic and material difficulties. Prolonged stress from any of these sources is often all it takes to damage health.

To think that the involvement of psychosocial processes in the relationship between income distribution and health means that we can forget about income distribution and concentrate on psy-chosocial interventions is the opposite of the truth. What it really means is that income distribution is an important determinant of the psychosocial welfare of a society. The importance of knowing that social cohesion is likely to be improved by narrower income differences is that it gives policy-makers a way of improving important aspects of the life of our society. Where people had previously only been able to throw their hands up in despair, it may now be possible to take practical steps to improve matters. Because income distribution is powerfully affected by government policy, governments may be able to improve the psychosocial condition and morale of the whole population.

STRESS AND HEALTH-RELATED BEHAVIOUR

One of the many ways in which psychosocial factors affect health is through health-related behaviour. A number of different kinds of behavioural health risks are likely to be influenced by general levels of social stress in the population. In a particularly revealing piece of research, Marsh showed that while smoking declined throughout the period 1976–90, it did so in each of the top three quartiles of the income distribution (the richest three-quarters of the population), but not among the poorest quarter (Marsh and McKay 1994). While the poorest quarter got relatively poorer (and some got absolutely poorer), their smoking increased. This was particularly apparent in the later 1980s when income differences widened particularly rapidly. It seems that smoking is now related to disadvantage not only when looking at the population in cross-section, but also when looking at changes over time. Despite the powerful financial disincentive to smoke, which might be expected to be strongest among the poorest, increased relative poverty and unchanged absolute incomes led the poor, against the national trend, to smoke more.

A more recent analysis of the Health and Lifestyles Survey in Britain found that while there was a clear socioeconomic gradient in success in giving up smoking, there was no gradient in the desire to give up (Jones 1995). As Marsh points out, giving up smoking is easier when your self-esteem is high, you feel optimistic about life and you feel in control. But when things are going badly and prospects look pretty hopeless, you are (as Hilary Graham has shown) more likely to regard smoking as your only relaxation and luxury – as well as wishing you could give up (Action on Smoking and Health 1993).

In an important sense, smoking has become a marker of socioeconomic stress. But there are signs of the same processes affecting other forms of behaviour which harm health. For example, among the many ways people respond to stress, unhappiness and unmet emotional needs, one is to increase their consumption of various comforting foods – which usually have high sugar and fat content – and of various drugs, including alcohol and of course tobacco. In its most extreme form, eating for comfort includes binge eating and bulimia. Once again, it is interesting to note that there were dramatic increases in the numbers of obese men and women of working age during the later 1980s while income differences were widening so rapidly (Department of Health 1993). It is easy to imagine that this may have been a result of increased unemployment and insecurity leading perhaps to decreased physical activity among dispirited people stuck at home eating for comfort.

The well-known tendency for people to start to eat more sweets when they give up smoking shows how sweets can function as alternative sources of comfort (Winkelstein and Feldman 1993). It is of course partly because smokers find it easier not to eat sweets that cigarette smoking has become particularly prevalent among younger women wanting to avoid putting on weight.

That people cling to various forms of 'unhealthy behaviour' while often wanting to give it up may seem suggestive of some driven, compulsive or addictive quality. To some extent they are attempts to satisfy what may be partly social needs. There are areas of consumption which exist in large part for their psychosocial effects. The desire for relaxants, disinhibitors, stimulants, etc. is presumably some indication of the psychosocial condition of the population. Alcohol has always been used throughout the population as a disinhibiter and to counter stress – particularly stress at social gatherings. It is also a relaxant. How much we feel we need it is shown by the amount consumed. Although well below average European Union levels, consumption in England and Wales is the equivalent of over a pint of beer a day for men over 16 years old and about half a pint for women (Institute for the Study of Drug Dependence 1994). Seven per cent of men and 2.5 per cent of women admit to getting drunk at least once a week. We saw in the last chapter that alcohol-related deaths were particularly closely related to income distribution internationally.

Before the decline in smoking, cigarettes had a social role which partly overlapped the social function of alcohol – people smoked to ease the social tensions of meetings and social gatherings. A cigarette was 'something to offer people'. Despite its long, slow decline, between a quarter and a third of British adults still smoke.

Some regard the amount of caffeine consumed in tea, coffee and soft drinks as another example of psychoactive consumption related to forms of stress. Estimates suggest that the average adult consumption is between 350 and 450 mg of caffeine per day – around twice the dose given when it is used medically as a stimulant.

As well as these self-prescribed comforters, there are the mood-altering drugs prescribed by general practitioners. Over 32 million prescriptions for various psychoactive drugs were dispensed for the population of England in 1994. Some, like Prozac, were designed to lift depression and make people feel happier about life; others, like the benzodizepines are intended to calm people and reduce anxiety. In addition, some of the illegal so-called 'recreational' drug-use should probably be seen as a response to similar problems. A number of illegal drugs were initially also regarded as easing social interaction: cannabis cigarettes were shared and believed by some – predictably in the 1960s – to be endowed with the power to transform human relations throughout society. Several of the more powerful drugs are valued particularly for inducing a sense of loss of ego and unity with others. According to Cameron and Jones, 'Our society not only needs tobacco, alcohol and other drugs of solace to relieve individuals of a great burden of pain and suffering but could not function in its present form without them' (Cameron and Jones 1985).

There is no doubt that we depend on a great many psychoactive props. It might have been thought that the need would decline as living standards rose – that eighteenth-century gin drinking reflected a desire to escape the material hardship and uncertainty of life – but the scale of the use of psychoactive drugs from all these various sources combined is probably as high as it has ever been. Although trends in smoking and in consumption of alcohol and caffeine differ from country to country, there is a widespread international growth in the use of illegal drugs and in psychoactive drugs provided by the pharmaceutical companies through the medical system. The pharmaceutical industry's ability to produce a range of psychoactive drugs is a fairly recent development and increased expenditure means that the consumption of them is very much more widespread than in any previous generation.

Given that the increasing use of the so-called 'talking therapies' might be seen as another response to similar psychological and emotional needs, it is interesting to note Gellner's explanation of the popularity and spread of the Freudian psychoanalytic theories which spawned them. Instead of dealing principally with the truth or falsity of Freudian theory, Gellner tries to explain why it became so popular (Gellner 1993). He argued that it filled a growing need. Suggesting that personal relationships became more problematic from the late nineteenth century, an attempt to provide a theoretical base for psychological therapy was bound to meet a popular demand.

There is also some evidence of more fundamental links than we normally recognise between stress and some of our common behavioural responses to it. Although we know that smoking, alcohol consumption and coffee are directly psychoactive, the tendency to eat sweet or fatty foods may have deeper roots than a purely neurotic need to give ourselves pleasure. There is a growing body of evidence which suggests that some of these foods may be marginally protective against some of the effects of stress. High cholesterol levels, which may result from eating for comfort, have been found to be associated with lower risk of injuries and suicides. A twenty-year follow-up study of 53,000 Swedish men and women found that men in the lowest 25 per cent of the distribution of cholesterol levels were almost three times as likely to die as a result of injuries. Most of these excess deaths were suicides. No similar pattern was found among women (Lindberg *et al.* 1992). Another study found lower cholesterol levels among cases of attempted suicide (Gallerani *et al.* 1995). A controlled trial which examined the behavioural effects of a low cholesterol diet involved feeding young monkeys diets which, although equally high in fat, were either high or low in cholesterol. The authors say that the animals given low-cholesterol diets 'were more aggressive and less affiliative' (Kaplan, J. R. *et al.* 1994). There are now a number of studies showing an association between low plasma cholesterol and higher risks of suicide, violence and accidents (Wardle 1995). It has been suggested that increased intake of sugars and fats when people feel low or depressed is a form of self-medication serving to relieve those feelings by increasing central serotonergic activity (Moller 1992).

There has always been a tendency among people working on behaviour and health to explain the higher levels of behavioural risks among the less well-off as a reflection of ignorance – or cost in the case of unhealthy food choices. The increased need for relaxants where socioeconomic stress is greatest has not been properly recognised and may be a major part of the explanation for the social distribution of some forms of health-damaging behaviour. We know that the consumption patterns associated with risk are often responses to various forms of stress and that several risky foodstuffs, as well as drink and tobacco, are psycho-active. Furthermore, epidemiological evidence shows that the years which saw the most rapid increase in relative poverty in the second half of the twentieth century also saw smoking increase among the poorest quarter of the population (Marsh and McKay 1994).

As well as suggesting an explanation for the social distribution of many behavioural health risks, this psychosocial perspective also helps to explain the resilience of the over consumption of various foods and drugs to the knowledge of their health consequences and the coaxings of health promoters. But perhaps more important than the social distribution of these things is the very high overall levels of consumption. Seen as a group, alcohol, cigarettes, the 32 million prescriptions for psychoactive drugs, caffeine-laden drinks and the comforting – probably antidepressant – sweet and fatty foods, present a picture of a remarkably neurotic society. Almost all of us know something both of the emotional and psychological gaps we use these things to plug, and of the difficulties of checking our own addictions – whether to chocolate, alcohol or anything else. They seem to indicate a fairly psychologically fragile society.

In the present context the social gradient in some behavioural risk factors may be more important for what it tells us about people's morale, stress and the extent to which they feel in control of their lives as for its direct impact on health. When thinking about the contribution of behavioural factors to social inequalities in health, it is important to bear four points in mind: that much the larger part of the social class gradient in heart disease is unexplained by behavioural risk factors; that if you get all the behavioural risk factors right, your most likely cause of death is still heart disease (Rose 1985); that diseases unrelated to smoking have as steep a social gradient as the ones that are related to smoking; and that there are class gradients in diseases for which we have no clear knowledge of behavioural risk factors. The distribution of behavioural risk factors in society does, however, suggest that psychosocial stress is greatest among the least well-off.

When thinking about the possible reasons for the high levels of consumption of psychoactive goods throughout society, there is an interesting point to do with blood pressure that it is perhaps worth keeping in the back of one's mind. In all societies except the earliest settled agriculturalists, nomadic herders, or hunters and gatherers, blood pressure tends to rise as people get older (Waldron *et al.* 1982). The more developed the society, the faster the rise of blood pressure with age seems to be. It has been suggested more than once that the tendency for blood pressure to rise is closely associated with the extent of a community's involvement in the market (Waldron *et al.* 1982; Eyer 1984). So thoroughly accepted and recognised is the tendency for blood pressure to rise as we get older, that doctors throughout the developed world always assess whether someone's blood pressure is high or low for their age. High blood pressure is nevertheless an important risk factor for common causes of death – such as stroke and heart disease. The odds against a dietary explanation of this phenomenon and for a psychosocial explanation were dramatically increased by a study which compared the age rise in blood pressure among a closed order of nuns with a control group of women. They found no age rise in blood pressure among the nuns. Because their control group was comparable in most other important respects, the authors concluded 'increased blood pressure in women . . . [during a span of] 20 years may be avoided by living in a stress-free monastic environment characterized by silence, mediation, and isolation from society' (Timio *et al.* 1988).

If it is plausible to see exposure to a number of behavioural risk factors as a response to social stress, and if it is right to think of social stress as having some societal causes (related to income distribution and social cohesion), then perhaps this partly explains Rose's observations (see chapter 2) that the proportion of people at high risk in any society results from a shift in the whole distribution of exposure to that risk factor, rather than from a change in the shape of the distribution (Rose 1992).

CONCLUSIONS

How does all this fit together? In the first part of this chapter we saw evidence from a variety of sources showing the potential of psychosocial processes to affect health directly. Many of the sources of psychosocial difficulties which we saw there are likely to be related to low relative income and to be more common in societies with low social cohesion. Most directly related to cohesion were the health effects of social networks and social participation.

In the second part of this chapter, we have seen how exposure to a number of health-related behavioural risk factors is likely to be increased in conditions of social stress, and how the high levels of exposure to less healthy lifestyles throughout the population may be an indication of a psychosocial vulnerability throughout society.

Although the effects of social networks on health may be powerful enough not to need to assume any other processes are involved, it seems likely that they are. There are almost certainly important effects of relative deprivation as well as broader effects of social cohesion. Indeed, within any society it is probably right to assume that the amount of social cohesion differs at different levels of society. Just as the poorest areas suffer more crime and more of a wide range of social problems, so it is likely that social cohesion is lower there than it is in middle-class neighbourhoods. Levels of social cohesion need not be regarded as a unitary factor with whole societies having high or low levels and little variation within them.

One attraction of placing some emphasis on this view was mentioned in chapter 6 above. Leon (personal communication) found that the causes of death which make an important contribution to the morality differences between Eastern and Western Europe are also the causes which are most important in terms of social class differences in mortality in Britain. Assuming that this means that there are some common causes for the two sets of differentials, it shortens the odds on social cohesion. The disintegration of public life and the decline into 'amoral familism' in Eastern Europe during the 1970s and 1980s is very clearly linked to the widening of the East–West mortality gap in those decades. Perhaps this is closer to the socially damaged nature of life in the run-down inner city areas in developed countries.

The material gleaned from social anthropology and social psychology in chapter 7 suggests the extent to which inequality and the associated lack of cohesion would prevent us experiencing ourselves as social beings. It may be that the epidemiology which shows the importance to health of close personal relations and wider social networks, is really showing a more fundamental way in which people need to live through and in relation to one another to find essential sources of self-confirmation.

The only half-way plausible approach to linking relative income to health without taking a psychosocial route, would be to suggest that in less egalitarian societies there are social pressures on consumption which mean that people are likely to divert expenditure from the satisfaction of the material preconditions for health. If it is felt necessary to have a smarter car and more expensive clothes, then expenditure may be diverted from food and other necessities. However, while there must be some effects of this kind, it would be difficult to make such an approach explain why the health gradient goes all the way up the social scale. The evidence of the strength of the impact which psychosocial factors can have on health removes much of the justification for preferring exclusively material pathways: so much so that it makes sticking to purely material explanations appear almost as a denial of the importance of the social.

In any estimation of the relative importance of different factors affecting population health, it is not simply the size of the additional health risk to exposed individuals which counts. It is also the proportion of the population exposed. Perhaps the consideration which above all others make psychosocial factors stand out as likely to be the most important determinants of population health in developed countries is simply the high proportion of the population exposed to various forms of psychosocial stress.

Chapter 10

Baboons, civil servants and children's height

Some of the most interesting work on the physiological pathways through which social organisation affects physical health comes, perhaps unexpectedly, from studies of other primates. It shows how position in the social hierarchy affects levels of stress and how chronic stress then affects central features of the ageing process.

For many years Robert Sapolsky has been studying wild baboons in the Serengeti and has shown some of the physiological effects of social dominance among them. He studies only adult males because 80 per cent of the females are pregnant or nursing and the anaesthetic darts he uses could endanger the pregnancies and disrupt the care of the young. He describes baboons as having to spend only about 4 hours a day foraging, leaving 12 hours a day for social behaviour. They have complicated social relations with patterns of dominance and subordination, alliances and friend-ships, and their competitiveness gives rise to a clearly defined social hierarchy. Sapolsky has shown that low-ranking males have much higher levels of glucocorticoids than high ranking ones, and has demonstrated that this is a response to the higher levels of stress experienced by subordinate animals as they are constantly faced down by more dominant ones (Sapolsky 1993). Glucocorticoids are steroid hormones released during stress as part of the 'fight or flight' mechanism. As such, they are a major component of the system by which the body's resources are diverted from non-urgent tasks, such as growth, tissue repair and the immune system, to preparing the body for immediate action and mobilising the necessary energy resources for muscles. The problem is not short bouts of stress produced by some temporary alarm, but the prolonged or chronic stress experienced by low-status animals which means that resources are withdrawn from health maintenance for long periods.

Central to the harmful effects of chronic stress is that the feedback mechanisms which regulate glucocorticoids become blunted by long-term exposure to raised levels during stress. Prolonged high glucocorticoid levels actually lead to the death of the neurone receptors in the hippocampus which are the basis of the feedback control system (Sapolsky 1992; Meaney *et al.* 1988). Low-status captive vervet monkeys collected and examined after death, were found not only to have multiple gastric ulcers and bite marks, but also significant hippocampal degeneration reflecting the neurodegeneration caused by continuous social stress and elevated glucocorticoids (Uno *et al.* 1989). With the passage of time, the blunting of the feedback mechanism causes a progressive rise in the basal levels of glucocorticoids. Among subordinate baboons glucocorticoid levels not only come to decline much more slowly following stressful events than they do among dominant baboons, but they also fail to decline to such a low level. (It is other parts of these same processes of chronic stress which were responsible for the changed size of the adrenal and thymus glands found in the bodies of paupers used in early anatomy lessons mentioned in the last chapter.) The whole system is gradually ratcheted up as the feedback mechanism is progressively damaged by higher levels of exposure. The result is that base levels of stress hormones tend to increase as we get older and the hippocampus suffers progressive damage. But as well as regulating glucocorticoids, the hippocampus is also particularly important in learning and memory. Hence a number of features of ageing, including memory loss, are likely to be related to the accumulated lifetime exposure to stress.

However, there is also evidence that responses to stress throughout adult life are affected by what happens early in life. It has been found that rats handled daily between birth and weaning have lower lifetime levels of stress and lower basal levels of glucocorticoids. Handling seems to make them more relaxed, so slowing down the vicious circle by which high levels of glucocorticoids damage the regulatory mechanism causing further rises. The differences between rats which are handled in early life and those which are not increases as they get older. The effects of hippocampal damage on brain function can be seen in the significantly better performance of the handled rats in learning to run mazes in later life (Meaney *et al.* 1988).

Several pathways by which prolonged social stress is likely to affect the health of low-status baboons have been demonstrated.

The elevated basal cortisol levels among low-status animals have been found to be associated with lower lymphocyte counts reflecting the suppressive effects of glucocorticoids on immunity. A number of studies (mentioned in the previous chapter) have demonstrated that human beings are also more likely to suffer from infections when under stress. A study was mentioned in the previous chapter which showed that the proportion of people who caught colds when given nasal drops containing cold viruses was related to stress levels (Cohen *et al.* 1991). Another study found that throat swabs taken from students during exams showed lower levels of immune functioning (Kennedy, S. *et al.* 1988).

The studies of baboons also showed that some risk factors for cardiovascular disease were also influenced by social status (Sapolsky 1993). Like the glucocorticoids, blood pressure in low-status animals also remained elevated for longer after a stressful encounter than it did among high-status animals. When it eventually declined, it did not decline to such low levels as were found among high-status animals. In humans this would increase the risk of heart disease and stroke among people lower down the social hierarchy. In addition, higher basal cortisol concentrations in low-status baboons were associated with a lower ratio of high-density to low-density lipoproteins. This leads to a more rapid accumulation of cholesterol deposits in the blood vessels, and the researchers reported a narrowing of the coronary artery and aorta in the low-status animals. In humans these changes are important risk factors for heart disease.

Brunner has drawn attention to a number of other similarities between the way risk factors for coronary heart disease are affected by social status among humans and baboons (Brunner 1996). He uses data from the two studies of 17,000 and 10,000 civil servants working in London. It was 'Whitehall I' which found age-adjusted death rates from heart disease four times as high among the most junior grades of office staff as among the most senior (see chapter 4). The second study was set up to take more detailed physiological and psychosocial measures in an effort to identify the source of the difference in health. Brunner reports that among civil servants, just as amongst the baboons, there were social gradients in levels of low-density lipoproteins (which increase the likelihood of clogged blood vessels and heart disease) and in high-density lipoproteins (which help clear cholesterol) – in both cases working to the disadvantage of the lower-status civil servants and baboons.

These, and differences in fibrinogen (which increases clotting), accounted for about one-third of the increased heart disease among low-ranking civil servants. Like Sapolsky, Brunner suggests a central role for chronic stress. He says that the most likely pathway 'links the chronic stress response of the hypothalamic pituitary adrenal system with resulting elevated levels of corticosteroids, to central obesity, insulin resistance, poor lipid profile and an increased tendency for the blood to clot' (Brunner 1996: p. 29). Although primarily concerned with coronary heart disease, Brunner also points out that similar pathways are likely to affect the immune system.

When discussing the similar physiological correlates of social status in humans and some other primates, it is important to emphasise that the relationship is not an expression of a sorting of the population according to genetic characteristics. Sapolsky established that the raised glucocorticoids are a direct response to social stress. He was able to observe the effects of wild animals moving to a new group where their social status changed, and of captive animals being placed in a different group. He also reported on the raised stress levels at times when the social hierarchy was unstable or when the whole group faced environmental challenges. Among baboons the raised stress seemed clearly related to the frequency of the challenge and threats from more dominant animals.

The fact that social hierarchy is negotiated in such different ways among humans compared to other primates should perhaps caution us against assuming that we are seeing the same basic processes in different species. Although people do face each other down and defer to those of higher status – and there are even reports of senior civil servants feeling physically sick after being verbally beaten up by bad-tempered government ministers – the underlying threat among humans is not of being bitten so much as of economic sanctions like losing your job or missing promotion. Brunner reported that the deteriorating ratio of high- to low-density lipo-proteins among low-status civil servants was significantly related to – amongst other things – the greater frequency of financial problems among them. But not only is it likely that low social status gives rise to increased stress for quite different reasons among human and other primate societies, but many of the causes of death related to low social status among humans do not exist among animals. For example, the causes of the large social class differences in childhood accidents is partly related to the lack of traffic-free play space and the more frequent sources of danger in poorer homes. Nor do stressed baboons take up drinking, smoking or drugs. But while bearing in mind the obvious important differences, it is worth remembering the common association of stress with lower social status.

THE HEIGHT AXIS

An important part of the way in which chronic stress translates socioeconomic inequality into health inequalities involves an intriguing story of the way emotional stress in childhood, height and social mobility are all related. Several crucial pieces of research have just been completed which cast an important new light on our understanding of the role played by height in health inequalities. It provides an interesting example of the interactions between socioeconomic factors, psychosocial processes and physiological and social outcomes.

It has been known for a long time that height is related to social mobility. Tall people move up the social scale and are more likely to get promotion than shorter people (Nystrom Peck 1992). It was shown as early as 1955 that taller women are more likely to marry up the social hierarchy than shorter women (Illsley 1955). In the Whitehall study it was found that the height of civil servants was more closely related to their position in the occupational hierarchy as adults than to the social class of their families as children (Marmot 1986). This suggests that the social sorting out, or selection by height, is even more powerful than the effect of social class on growth during childhood.

For a long time it was assumed that the explanation of why tall people were more likely to move up the social scale was that everyone else somehow looked up to and respected taller people, as if they had a natural superiority. However, an important breakthrough came in a paper from Montgomery, Bartley et al. (1996). They used data from a large study which has followed up a cohort of 17,000 people since they were born in 1958. Information on whether or not they were unemployed in early adulthood was used as an indicator of people's likely occupational mobility. They found that, although the chances of being unemployed were – as expected – greater among shorter people, unemployment was much more likely among people who had been short as children than among those who were short adults. The data showed very clearly that unemployment in adulthood was much more closely related to height at age 7 than to adult height. (Although heights at each age are closely related, people grow at different speeds so that not all short 7 year olds become short adults, nor all tall 7 year olds tall adults.)

This important finding forces a fundamental reappraisal of what is going on, and it is all the more important because it has always been clear that height is also very closely related to health. Here the assumed explanation seemed to be that taller people were simply better physical specimens all round. But if tall people were upwardly mobile because everyone was impressed by their physical presence, then their social mobility would have been most closely related to adult height. That it turns out to be more closely related to height in childhood means that adult height is merely a distant reflection of something in childhood which affects both childhood height and future social mobility. The two questions which then arise are: what are the determinants of childhood height? And, are any of them plausible influences on social mobility later in life?

In poor societies, nutrition is no doubt one of the most important factors. However, as standards of nutrition improve during the course of economic development, it is likely that it becomes less important as an explanation of the remaining differences in height in richer countries. As well as environmental influences, we should also remember that there is a large genetic component tending to make heights of children more like the heights of their parents. What is interesting is that several recent pieces of research in developed countries have shown that psychosocial and emotional factors also have an important influence on height. A Swedish study which asked adults about their childhood conditions found that in addition to shorter people being brought up in economic hardship and having larger families, they were also more likely to have suffered domestic conflict in childhood (Nystrom Peck and Lundberg 1995).

Using data from the 1958 cohort study which, unlike the Swedish study, did not rely on retrospective recall, Power found that shortness in adulthood was associated with reports of psycho-social problems in childhood – particularly bed-wetting (Power and Manor 1995). Bed-wetting is always regarded as a sign of emotional disturbance. Most recently, Montgomery and Bartley also used data from the 1958 birth cohort study to prove conclusively that slow growth in childhood was associated with family conflict (Montgomery and Bartley, forthcoming 1996). Parental height was used to control for the important genetic influences on height.

What is new is the evidence that psychosocial factors contribute even to the variations in height around the normal range. A condition called 'psychogenic dwarfism', in which children cease to grow, has long been recognised to result from severe emotional trauma in childhood. But this was regarded as an extreme effect. It was frequently recognised that short children often had emotional difficulties, but these were usually assumed to be the result, rather than the cause, of being short (Stabler and Underwood 1986).

An isolated report soon after the Second World War suggested that psychosocial factors had an important effect on normal growth rates (Widdowson 1951). The study was designed to assess the effect of nutrition on growth. It was decided to supplement the rather meagre dietary rations provided in German orphanages soon after the war. Growth of children in one orphanage where children were given additional food was compared with the growth of children in another who got only the basic rations. However a changeover in the matrons running the orphanages halfway through the study appeared to have a bigger effect on growth than the nutritional supplementation. Growth was fastest wherever the warm, affectionate matron was, and slower in the presence of a colder, undemonstrative and more authoritarian matron. In this context the longstanding tendency to regard all the associations between shortness and emotional difficulties in children as the emotional consequences of being short is particularly interesting. Montgomery outlines a possible physiological pathway which could explain how psychosocial factors impact on height (Montgomery and Bartley, forthcoming 1996). He points out that frequent sleep disturbance would reduce the secretion of growth hormone, and also suggests that stress can lead to raised levels of beta-endorphin which inhibits the release of growth hormone in pre-pubertal children. Studies of rhesus monkeys have also shown that growth hormone release is affected by the quality of mother–child bonding (Champoux et al. 1989).

We can now see not only that height is influenced by psychosocial factors during childhood, but also that these same psychosocial factors are likely to explain the greater occupational success and upward social mobility of taller people. Basically they are taller because they have escaped some of the emotional trauma and psychological stress (often resulting from family conflict) which other children have suffered, and they are more likely to be upwardly mobile during their working lives because they are in better emotional and psychological shape than shorter people. Their greater emotional security probably means that they fit in better and function better.

The use of parental height to control for genetic influences on height is important. Twin studies suggest that in developed societies genes explain a much larger proportion of the differences in height than they do of most other important developmental and health variables. As much as 80 per cent of the variations in height may be due to genetic inheritance. If this were all we knew, it would seem likely that the part of social mobility which is selective for height would amount to a form of genetic selection. However, because these pieces of research control for the genetic component, and have identified a specific environmental determinant of height as related to social mobility, we can say with some confidence that this is not evidence to suggest that this is a mechanism for the selection of genetically superior tall people. It is interesting to note in this context that the environmental component of the variance in height is, like health, also related to income distribution. As we noted in chapter 5, Steckel found that differences in the average heights of populations were related to income distribution (Steckel 1983; 1994).

The question then arises as to why height is a good proxy for health later in life. What makes taller people healthier? Part of the answer is undoubtedly because their advantage in terms of social mobility means that they live in better – and less stressful – conditions, but they are healthier even after controlling for their social class or occupational status (Marmot *et al.* 1984; Marmot 1986; Nystrom Peck 1992). However, as well as the important influence of their current circumstances, there are reasons for thinking that the psychosocial processes linking childhood height to adult social mobility will also make a direct contribution to the greater healthiness of taller people.

A Japanese study compared levels of cognitive functioning among twins in later life – when they were between 50 and 78 years old (Hayakawa *et al.* 1992b). The researchers used tests of cognitive functioning which are particularly sensitive to the gradual decline in mental ability which goes with ageing. The average test scores in this study therefore deteriorated with age: scores were lower among the twins in their sixties than among those in their fifties, and were lower still among those in their seventies. In fact, most of the twins were in their fifties and sixties and many had had their childhood disrupted by the Second World War. Some had lost parents or been adopted, and it was this misfortune which provided a special opportunity for research. The aim of the study was to see how the cognitive functioning of each twin differed from that of his or her twin pair. (The study was restricted to same-sex twins.) How alike or different twins were from each other could then be analysed, not only according to whether they were genetically identical or non-identical, but according to how much of their childhood they spent together. The results showed two important things. First, the fact that cognitive functioning was as alike among pairs of non-identical twins as it was among identical twins on two of the three tests, showed that cognitive functioning in later life is determined largely by environmental rather than genetic factors. (Any genetic component of the similarity should have increased the similarity between the identical twins.) Second, the study showed that each twin's score was much more like his or her partner's if they had lived together throughout childhood (whether or not they were identical). The earlier they were separated, the less alike was their cognitive functioning in later life. Correlations rose from around 0.1 among twins separated between 0 and 5 years old to around 0.7 among those who remained together throughout their childhood (see figure 10.1). This provides very powerful evidence that the decline in cognitive functioning in later life is strongly influenced by what happens in early life. (It is also an important exception to the work of Plomin, which discounts the importance of the shared childhood environment in influencing many developmental measures (Plomin and Daniels 1987; Dunn and Plomin 1991).

This pattern is clearly reminiscent of the research, summarised earlier in this chapter, on the beneficial effect of stroking young animals early in life (Sapolsky 1992). Experiments showed that handled animals had lower levels of chronic stress and so advanced more slowly into the vicious spiral by which raised cortisol levels damaged the hippocampus and hastened the decline in cognitive functioning with ageing.

The implication is that cognitive functioning of ageing Japanese twins was more alike if they spent their childhood together because they would then have shared more of the same emotional

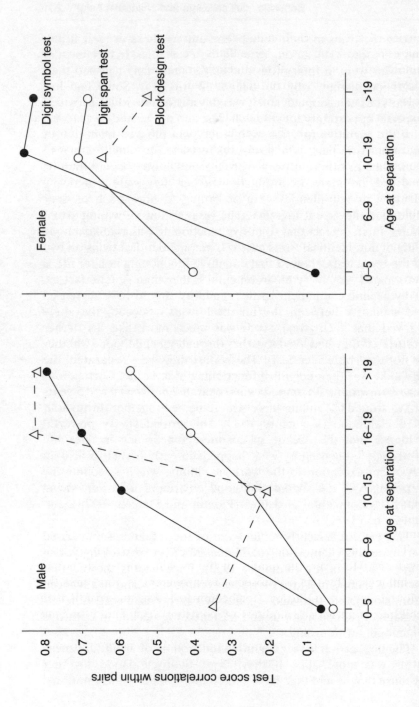

Figure 10.1: The decline of mental ability in later life is strongly affected by childhood environment. On these tests of cognitive functioning elderly identical twins were more like each other if they had spent more of their childhood together.
Source: Hayakawa 1992b.

environment. Like the handled rats which were better at learning mazes in their rat old age, some twins had shared an experience of emotional warmth, physical affection and security, and so had a slower decline in cognitive functioning in later life. Others shared a less emotionally supportive and secure beginning and so shared an earlier mental decline in later life.

But it is not merely the decline in cognitive functioning in old age which has been linked into this process. Presumably the tall, emotionally secure, upwardly socially mobile people, would have had lower stress levels throughout life. Though still affected by stressful circumstances, they were likely to have been less vulnerable than others. Lower stress responses would in turn mean less of the health-damaging effects of stress relayed through either the immune or endocrine systems (Sapolsky 1994). With the body geared for 'fight or flight' less often, more time and resources would have been devoted to the claims of the immune system, growth and tissue repair.

Linking the work of Bartley, Montgomery and Power on the 1958 British birth cohort, to that of Sapolsky and his colleagues who have identified some of the most important endocrine and neurological pathways through which psychosocial influences affect health, and linking that to Hayakawa's study of cognitive ageing in twins, we arrive at a fairly clear indication of why taller people are upwardly mobile, are healthier and live longer. Stress levels early in life (as indicated by things such as family conflict and bed-wetting) reduce growth and affect stress responses throughout much of life. People who were brought up in a less emotionally secure environment as children are likely to suffer higher levels of stress as adults. Their chances of moving up through the occupational hierarchy, their social functioning and their health are damaged by their sense of insecurity and its emotional consequences.

This sounds like rather a lot to hang on comparatively little evidence. However, the quality of the evidence that early height is influenced by the psychosocial environment is good and the Montgomery and Bartley (forthcoming, 1996) study of British children confirms the findings of Nystrom Peck and Lundberg (1995) in Sweden, and of Widdowson's (1951) work in German orphanages. Nor is there much doubt, at least among animals, about the benefits of increased physical contact early in life. It has been shown to affect growth hormone in infancy (Champoux *et al.*

1989) as well as stress levels and cognitive functioning later in life (Meany *et al.* 1988; Sapolsky 1992; Hayakawa 1992b). Without these links it would be extremely difficult to explain why adult social mobility should be more closely related to childhood height than adult height. These connections also make good sense of findings such as Power's that the best predictor of health in early adulthood available in the 1958 birth cohort (National Child Development Study) was teachers' assessments of children's behavioural problems when they were 16 years old (Power *et al.* 1991). It also makes good sense of what is known about the lasting effects on child development of family conflict. It might also provide part of the explanation of why some of the evaluations of pre-school education have shown major benefits in terms of better employment and lower involvement in crime when children reach adulthood (Schweinhart and Weikart 1993). Lastly, it should caution people against taking the relationship between measures of mental ability in childhood and achieved social mobility in adult life as evidence that social mobility is a reflection of innate intelligence (Saunders 1996).

The fact that childhood influences on later life are important does not of course mean that the lives people lead as adults, and the circumstances in which they live, do not also exert a powerful influence on health. We saw plenty of examples in the last chapter of the health impact of psychosocial circumstances in adult life. The Japanese twin study shows that there is plenty of room (unexplained variance) for influences from circumstances experienced later in life.

Regardless of whether a society is supportive or not, those who succumb to its various difficulties will usually be the most vulnerable. That it is frequently possible to find evidence of individual vulnerability among those who fair least well does not mean that the numbers failing will not be dramatically influenced by the rigours or supportivness of the socioeconomic environment. The tendency for those who are most vulnerable to succumb first – in this or any other area – does not absolve the current circumstances in which people live from their share of the blame. Even if everyone who succumbs to some environmental difficulty also had some individual vulnerability factor, this does not mean that a change in the harshness of the socioeconomic environment might not halve or double the members who succumb.

The relationship between height in childhood and social mobility in adulthood is an important contributor to the volume of health-related social mobility which was discussed in chapter 4. Its size is however limited by two factors. One is that the better health of the tall is not simply the better prognosis they grow up with: it is also the result of the better conditions in which they are placed as adults by their upward social mobility. The second factor is that there is a very steep social gradient in psychosocial or emotional welfare in young children. When discussing in chapter 8 the decline in reading standards in primary schools which took place in the later 1980s while relative poverty increased, we mentioned findings from a study of 15,000 children whose development has been followed since their birth in 1970. In an assessment carried out when they were 10 years old, it was found that rates of hyperactivity were over three times as high, and conduct disorders four times as high, in social class V (unskilled manual occupations) as in social class I (professional occupations). Differences in anxiety were less than twofold. The data, taken from Woodroffe *et al.* (1993), are shown in figure 10.2. Rather than showing that part of the process of social mobility is selective for health, the very heavy preponderance of these kinds of problems among young children in poorer circumstances is probably an important indication of why rates of social mobility are not higher than they are. The links we have described must be an important reason for much of the additional educational and career disadvantages suffered by children from poorer homes. Despite all the difficulties of quantification and measurement and the uncertainty about exactly what one should be trying to measure, the gradients in behavioural and emotional problems shown in figure 10.2 testify to the enormous burden which the growing rates of deprivation among families with children impose not only on the children themselves but on society at large for decades to come.

Height is not the only evidence of a link between early emotional experience and health in adulthood. In a study of over 5,000 children born in 1946, Wadsworth showed that the emotional impact of family disruption exerted a powerful influence on health and social functioning in early adulthood (Wadsworth 1984). People whose parents had divorced, died or permanently separated were more likely to suffer from stomach ulcers or colitis and psychiatric illness by the time they were 26 years old. Their marriages were also more likely to end in separation or divorce, and they were more likely to have convictions for sexual and

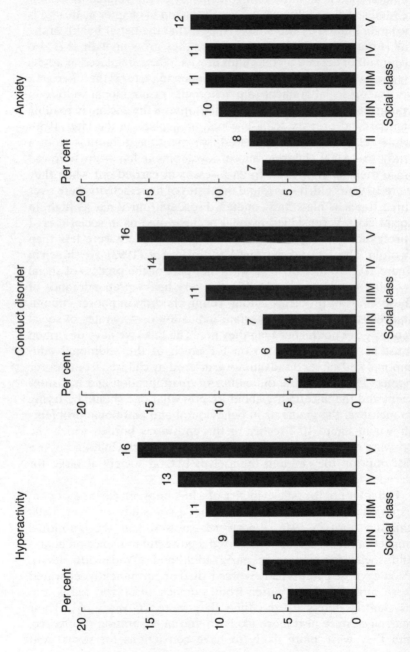

Figure 10.2: Behaviour problems age 10 years: social class, Great Britain 1980
Source: A. Osborn, data from the British 1970 birth cohort, as quoted in Woodroffe *et al.* 1993

violent offences – even after controlling for birth order, family size and social class. They were also less likely to have good relationships with their own children. Once again, these effects of emotional stress are more strongly associated with family disruption occurring early in childhood. In this study the effects were larger in the 0–5 age group than among those over 5.

As well as relating height to family dissension in childhood, Lundberg found that illness in a study population aged between 30 and 75 was closely related to family dissension even after controlling for social class (Lundberg 1993). Mortality risks were over 50 per cent higher for those who had experienced family conflict in childhood.

The psychosocial influences on health, height and social mobility do not come into the picture instead of material and economic factors: they are rather one of the pathways that explain how material factors influence these outcomes, and why factors like health, height and social mobility are related to social class. If the aim is to improve the welfare of populations, it would be unwise to try to treat the psychosocial symptoms without reducing the underlying scale of relative deprivation. Not only are the two hard to separate even in individual cases, but the provision of any kind of service on a scale large enough to make an impact on these problems in society as a whole would be totally unrealistic: there is little evidence of effectiveness even on a small scale, and the cost of such an approach on a societal scale would be entirely prohibitive.

Part V

Redistribution, economic growth and the quality of life

Chapter 11

Social capital: putting Humpty together again

Too often life seems dominated by economics, and it looks as if this book is about how it dominates even the length of life. But more fundamentally it is about the importance of human social needs, and the way health is affected by the growing conflict between economic systems and the fulfilment of our social needs. Its main message is of the primary importance of social relations to us as social beings. At all stages in human societies, whether rich or poor, the quality of social relations has been a prime determinant of human welfare and the quality of life.

As the powerful logic of the market extends its tentacles ever wider, it is easy to think of economics as a mental illness which leads to the perception of all human behaviour as springing from an egotistical desire to maximise consumption. While we are all aware that there is life outside the marketplace, I remember an economist who was more than usually aware of how much economics left out. His response was to build models which extended beyond the monetary economy. He used a technique called input–output analysis which attempts to summarise all transactions in an economy by tabulating what every industry buys from, and sells to, every other industry. In one study he tried not only to take into account environmental factors, by building in an ecological table of transactions in the natural world, but also our social interactions. This involved a table covering what went on between households. Along with a new battery of social commodities to be traded which included things like 'respect', one of the things he decided human beings need from each other was love. This was therefore included in the table of things traded, along with sheet steel, plastics and electronic instruments. He then realised that people not only want to receive love, they want to give it as well. This gave rise to two separate social goods which could be traded: 'love received' and 'love tendered'. The distinction between tradable commodities and relations of love and respect which are antipathetic to market exchange was overlooked.

The social and health effects of larger income differences provide a powerful reason for reducing them. Greater equality has traditionally been a socialist aim. But even among those who continue to advocate it, we find their rationale has been infected by the logic of economic relations. Greater income equity was originally seen as a way of furthering social harmony and reducing the structural basis for conflict between people: so much so that the same aspiration was also expressed in the socialist practice of referring to their fellows as 'brother' or 'sister'. But increasingly, income redistribution has been advocated – not for how it might benefit social relations – but simply as a demand for a fairer share-out of goods and services among societies assumed to be made up of self-interested individuals. This change is an important indication of how far economic ideology has penetrated: even those who at least partly reject the market have lost sight of our social core and unwittingly translated the socialist aims to fit a marketised humanity. The uninspiring vision is, at best, of a competitive, de-socialised equality.

The evidence reviewed in the preceding chapters cannot be easily dismissed. Income distribution has been shown by eight different groups of researchers to be related to national mortality rates in various groups of developed and less developed countries on ten separate sets of data (see chapter 5). It cannot be regarded as the result of one or two chance findings. Some people may suspect that it should be explained as the spurious expression of some underlying relationship – resulting from something that separately affects both income distribution and health. While income distribution is likely to serve as a measure of closely related features of society such as social cohesion, the possibilities of the relationship being a spurious reflection of some wholly different intervening variable are extremely remote. There are several major difficulties facing that line of thought. First, the statistical relationship between income distribution and national mortality rates is strong: correlations of 0.6, 0.7 or 0.8 are reported. Normally the correlations between them and any supposed intervening variable would have to be stronger, so the search would have to be for something more closely related to both income distribution and mortality than that. We know of nothing that would fit. Not only that, but it would have to fit when looking at the relationship cross-sectionally – independently among developed countries and less developed countries; it would have to fit when looking at changes over time among developed countries; and finally it would have to fit when looking at the relationship between income distribution and mortality within countries, both among fifty states in the USA and among small areas of Britain (Kaplan *et al.* 1996; Kennedy *et al.* 1996; Ben Shlomo *et al.* 1996). This is an impossibly tall order.

On top of that, it is known that areas of public expenditure such as housing and medical care do not exert an influence on population health anywhere near powerful enough to explain this relationship, even if they were related to it. Statistical analysis has shown, however, that controlling for total government expenditure or expenditure just in areas such as these does not remove the relationship. In this context another contrast between Sweden and Japan is interesting. While very alike in terms of their narrow income distributions and high life expectancy, they arc dramatically different – not only in relation to family structure as we pointed out in chapter 8 – but also in relation to the proportion of GNP taken in government social expenditure. In Sweden government social expenditure is a higher proportion of GNP than in any other OECD country; in Japan it is lower than in any other OECD country (Hills 1994). Nor is the relationship removed when controlled for GNPpc, average incomes, absolute poverty, race or smoking (see chapter 5).

We saw in chapter 6 that societies which are both egalitarian and healthy are also markedly more socially cohesive than others. Above all, the public sphere in these societies seemed to be incorporated in social life rather than being abandoned to the negative market relations between self-interested households – Banfield's so-called 'a-moral familism' (Banfield 1958). With reduced income inequality, people are connected in public life through a variety of social organisations, purposes and activities. Some sense of the moral collectivity and of social purpose remains important. In chapter 8 we saw the typical symptoms which appear when inequality increases and social divisions become deeper. As well as higher death rates from most causes, these societies tend to show markedly higher rates of alcohol-related deaths, accidents, homicide, crime, violence and probably drug use. As a set of social problems, the statistical connection between them and wider social divisions is very plausible. They are very much what one might expect symptoms of greater socioeconomic stress to be.

Looking at the epidemiological and physiological evidence of how greater socioeconomic inequality could affect physical health, it is clear that there is no shortage of possible pathways. Chapters 9 and 10 show that there is very firm evidence that psychosocial processes can exert a major influence on health. Not only do many of the psychosocial associations with health show stronger correlations than those between material factors and health (certainly on a population attributable risk basis), but the fact that they do so is consistent with the interpretation of the epidemiological transition put forward in chapter 3.

So what are the implications of this picture? Some people would rather the relationship between income distribution and health were explained in terms of the absolute material deprivation of the poor. Believing in the importance of material factors, some feel that a psychosocial explanation belittles and psychologises the relationship. In fact it makes it much more important and raises much more fundamental issues. First, in terms of how much it matters. If health were being damaged by objective material factors, regardless of their social connotations, it would have few wider implications. Assuming that the last decade has been an exception, and that 'trickle-down' is normally part of economic growth, problems of absolute material poverty would be expected to solve themselves in the normal course of economic growth. The fact that health inequalities have widened in Britain during most of the second half of the twentieth century and in the USA and France for varying periods suggests that these problems do not solve themselves.

From the point of view of the experience of people involved, if health is being damaged as a result of psychosocial processes, this matters much more than it would if the damage resulted from the immediate physical effects of damp housing or poor quality diets. If it were not for the psychosocial effects we are talking about, it would be possible to eat a diet with too many chips and too much fried food and be perfectly happy. The same would be true of smoking and taking too little exercise. In terms of the practical problems they produce, damp homes can involve extra work and a good deal of frustration. If these were the major causes of health inequalities and the explanation of the relationship between health and income distribution, then it would not be so far from the truth to say that life for the relatively poor might be shorter, but perhaps not much less sweet, than it was for the rich. But this problem is important because that is so far from the truth. To feel depressed, cheated, bitter, desperate, vulnerable, frightened, angry, worried about debts or job and housing insecurity; to feel devalued, useless, helpless, uncared for, hopeless, isolated, anxious and a failure: these feelings can dominate people's whole experience of life, colouring their experience of everything else. It is the chronic stress arising from feelings like these which does the damage. It is the social feelings which matter, not exposure to a supposedly toxic material environment. The material environment is merely the indelible mark and constant reminder of the oppressive fact of one's failure, of the atrophy of any sense of having a place in a community, and of one's social exclusion and devaluation as a human being.

In terms of the quality of life, which is ultimately a matter of people's subjective sense of well-being, the psychosocial processes round inequality, social cohesion and its effect on health, are overwhelmingly important. They are important not only from the point of view of those low down the social scale who suffer them most, but also because the deterioration of public life, the loss of a sense of community, and particularly the increase in crime and violence, are fundamentally important to the quality of life for everyone.

To say that factors related to income distribution are so important to the real subjective quality of life across society as a whole contrasts with the common tendency to regard the quality of life as almost synonymous with the material standard of living. In chapter 3 we looked at the changing relationship between economic growth and increases in life expectancy. As noted there, there are reasons for thinking that health is a better guide to the quality of life than measures of real income and GNPpc. While economic measures are largely confined to quantitative material change, health is sensitive to material and social circumstances and is affected by qualitative and quantitative change. Its sensitivity to the dominating psychosocial quality of life means that health has a strong claim to be a more reliable indicator of the quality of life than the various economic indices. Although we might assume that more meant better at almost any level of wealth, if everything else remained equal, we know that social and environmental considerations do not remain equal: GNPpc is a poor guide to the subjective quality of life.

One of the reasons for the continued interest in economic growth is a belief that every individual's desire for increased income can be summed into a societal desire for increased income. But given what we know about the power of income distribution and the importance of relative rather than absolute income, it is possible that this is based on a false assumption. Perhaps the individual desire for increased income is primarily a desire to have the things richer people have and to occupy the social position of richer people: that is to say, it may be primarily a desire to increase one's relative income. The advantages of being richer are, after all, most clearly demonstrated by the rich in one's own society. The desire to win millions of pounds is presumably a desire to be one of the rich and to have their freedom and command over resources. It may be a long way from a desire to be part of a society with a larger GNPpc. Indeed, some less well-off people might prefer to be relatively better-off people in a poorer society.

The other politically persuasive reason for pursuing economic growth is that faster growth rates are associated with reductions in unemployment, a decrease in income insecurity and with increases in business profits. But these are in a sense merely welcome by-products of the growth process. To want continuous growth in order to solve problems of that kind is merely a form of addiction: during the economic highs the problems are temporarily solved only to return in the next recession. The problems which the economic upturns seem to solve need a more fundamental and durable solution which would hold even in the absence of growth.

The idea that the interests of the poor are the primary moral justification for economic growth in the developed world has worn thin in the face of the evidence that the growth of the last decade or so has been accompanied more by a process of trickle-up than trickle-down. However, now it is clear that the main problems of poverty (at least within the developed world) are problems of relative poverty, we know that they have to be faced directly: we can no longer make the complacent assumption that they will disappear as we all get richer together.

In chapter 3 we discussed how rising life expectancy might be related to economic growth. We saw that if there had been fully quality-adjusted price indices to use in the preparation of the data illustrated in figure 3.1, it would have moved countries to the right with the passage of time. While this could have brought together the rising part of each curve, it would also have meant that there was even less relationship between GNPpc and life expectancy among the rich countries at any point in time: the flat part of the cross-sectional curve would have become flatter as it was stretched out further to the right.

We were left looking for an explanation of why the horizontal part of the curve of life expectancy rises with the passage of time. The only explanation suggested in chapter 3 was that new knowledge, new technology, new goods and services made a difference to health and shifted the curve upwards over time. It was argued that differences in the rate at which these innovations diffused among the populations of the developed countries may have little relationship to growth rates and GNPpc. Thus once a threshold level of development has been achieved, so that basic necessities are assured and societies have bought their way into modern technology, the differences between them are relatively unimportant. In so far as societies are part of the international market, they will enjoy the fruits of innovation (and probably contribute to them) regardless of their measured income growth.

In terms of the growing concern with the likely environmental consequences of economic growth (but see Beckerman 1995) and the demands for 'zero growth', the discussion in chapter 3 leads us to a useful distinction. In terms of resource shortages and pollution, the main threat comes from the quantitative component of growth, from using more resources, more energy and producing more waste. Growth from qualitative improvements not only produces benefits which raise fewer problems, but the process of innovation from which they arise may be made to serve environmental purposes. Already a large component of innovation is resource saving and this tends to reduce waste. Even where such savings are not made, design improvements often add to the use-value of goods without changing resource costs. This holds out the possibility that we could have something close to zero growth (as currently measured), but continue to enjoy the fruits of design improvements and innovations focused more rigorously on serving the environment and consumer. In other words, it is possible to envisage continued improvements in the material standard of living which are not bought at the expense of the environment. Growth which was zero in purely quantitative terms would not mean putting up with our current messy material infrastructure, compromised technology and way of life for the rest of human existence. We can have innovation without growth.

If we balk at the attempt to use qualitative technical change to explain chapter 3's puzzling problem of ever higher horizontal curves relating GNPpc to life expectancy, then there seems to be only one other remotely plausible explanation of it. As the two explanations are compatible, we can take whatever mix of them we choose. The additional explanation depends on the loose links between economic development and the processes of cultural and psychosocial change.

One of the most important advantages of higher living standards is the increased sense of security and the slow disappearance of the more brutal aspects of life. Historically speaking, there is perhaps a gradual softening of different aspects of social and emotional life as living standards rise. Among the most obvious signs of this process are things like the abolition of capital punishment in many countries and the abolition of corporal punishment in schools. Changes in child-rearing practices illustrate these processes more clearly than some. DeMause begins the introductory chapter of his *History of childhood* saying: 'The history of childhood is a nightmare from which we have only recently begun to awaken. The further back in history one goes, the lower the level of child-care, and the more likely children are to be killed, abandoned, beaten, terrorized and sexually abused' (DeMause 1974, p. 1). He suggests that if we go back far enough, 'most children were what we would now consider abused' (ibid., p. 3). DeMause goes as far as to suggest that 'the central force for change in history is neither technology nor economics, but the psychogenic changes in personality occurring because of successive generations of parent–child interactions.' He believed that this process 'placed definite limits on what could be achieved in all other spheres' of life (ibid., p. 3).

Rather than agreeing with deMause's assertion of the autonomy and primacy of changes in child-rearing, it would seem more reasonable to regard them as part of the civilising effect of economic development. Given the importance of the childhood emotional environment to people's later development and health (which we saw in chapter 10), we would expect the improvements in child-rearing to have produced major physical and mental benefits during the rest of life. But the changes in childhood were, of course, part of the more general social development of society which has affected people of all ages. The profound psychosocial changes are perhaps clearest when we remind ourselves of how much of pre-industrial and early industrial life now seems barbaric to us. The way any society treats its law breakers, its mentally handicapped and its poor tells us a lot about the progress of that society's humanity. Abandoning the branding of beggars, the burning of witches and the public execution or hanging of criminals reflects an important psychological transformation.

Given the importance of psychosocial influences on health (discussed in chapters 9 and 10), then the decline of fear and insecurity and the increasing air of tolerance in society are important. The fact that we sometimes fail to recognise both the importance and existence of these immaterial cultural developments does not disprove their existence. The growing social tolerance has continued, not without reversals, during the second half of the twentieth century. Changes such as the legalisation of homosexuality and of abortion have reduced the occasions for fear: the fear of arrest and imprisonment for homosexuals and the fear of social stigmatisation among young women who become pregnant before marriage. These, together with the introduction of modern contraceptive methods, have changed sexuality from a furtive, highly repressed and fearful activity, into something which may one day emerge as a relaxed expression of our humanity. Rather than just affecting young people, these changes have led to a decrease in repression and the development of more tolerant attitudes round sexuality throughout life.

The ending of compulsory military service has presumably reduced people's familiarity with some forms of brutality. In social relations more generally there has been a widespread move towards preferring more familiar forms of address and the abandonment of some of the signs of deference and servitude between social classes. An indication of how much more aware than our predecessors we are of the importance of emotional life is perhaps shown by the recognition of post-traumatic stress disorder among people working in the emergency services. The growing attempts to provide counselling for people who have had to cope with harrowing situations contrast starkly with the normality of such experiences in earlier centuries.

The concept of 'civilisation' comes close to capturing the most important kinds of cultural and psychosocial change which accompany economic growth. It incorporates the necessary notions of human dignity and emancipation – both social and material emancipation. Although civilisation is not the same as economic growth, it appears to be one of the forms in which we take the benefits of material progress. That it has a major cultural and ideological component means that it is only loosely related to growth. As well as dignity and emancipation, the word 'civilisation' contains the notion of civility and conjures up ideas of citizenship and the nature of social development. It comes close to the issues of social cohesion discussed in chapter 7. Certainly, life in societies with wider income distributions seems less civilised. Yet, despite the concept being far from synonymous with the notion of economic growth, there is in everyone's minds a recognition that civilisation has its material aspects: the public health measures introduced in late Victorian Britain were emancipating and clearly made life more civilised. Standards of civilisation are widely shared in developed societies and, as they progress with the passage of time, they could perhaps provide part of the 'income-gearing factor' which raises the curve of life expectancy from one period to the next.

The attraction of giving space to this kind of explanation is not merely that the data are difficult to explain any other way. It is also that it begins to provide a more unified view of the major influences on health both as it changes over time internationally and as it is affected by the degree of equality and social cohesion within societies. We need to put together a combination of what is summed up in the notions of social cohesion and civilisation. If we could use a dose of egalitarianism to turn the idea of civilisation into an inclusive rather than an exclusive concept, we would perhaps have an idea of the social conditions for health. The result would be close to something we might call human dignity. Given that there are emancipating as well as belittling and corrosive aspects of material advance, such a concept serves to combine some (but not all) features of economic growth with the psychosocial progress which accompanies them. But the importance of the concept of civilisation lies beyond health: as a result of the psychosocial pathways which relate material life to health, we would expect that the social conditions for health would also be indicative of the quality of life. We end up with a concept of the quality of life which is a little more distanced from economic growth and aligned with something closer to an amalgam of civilisation and social cohesion.

We can perhaps only hint at its content. From epidemiological research we can take social affiliations and social support, a sense of control and of security. In addition, social cohesion relates easily to the sense of coherence which Antonovsky and others have suggested is protective of health (Antonovsky 1992; Lundberg and Nystrom Peck 1994). Although he regarded it as something individuals either had or did not have, it might be better in the present context to see a sense of coherence as a property of social groups and societies. Given a basis of social justice founded in narrower income differences and in full civil rights, there will be fewer fault-lines in the 'moral community'. Antonovsky's 'sense of coherence' requires that individuals have a sense of purpose and role which, for most people, can only be secure if it has wider support from a shared ideology and system of values. If there is not a sense of social justice, then the legitimacy of social institutions is fundamentally weakened and the moral community which makes social life coherent is lacking. Cohesion and coherence are therefore likely to closely related to social justice.

Putnam, whose work on the strength of civic society in the regions of Italy we discussed in chapter 6, uses the concept of 'social capital'. He says:

> By 'social capital' I mean features of social life – networks, norms, and trust – that enable participants to act together more effectively to pursue shared objectives. . . . To the extent that the norms, networks, and trust link substantial sectors of the community and span underlying social cleavages – to the extent that the social capital is of a bridging sort – then the enhanced cooperation is likely to serve broader interests and to be widely welcomed.
>
> (Putnam 1995, pp. 664–5)

It is interesting that although Putnam very reasonably ascribes the decline in social participation in the United States to the growth of television, he clearly sees bridging social cleavages as a crucial function of social capital. Given that social cleavages would be easier to bridge if they were smaller, this contrasts rather starkly with the lack of attention he gives to the influence of income distribution on social cohesion.

People in the developed countries have become increasingly aware of the contrast between the material success and social failure of modern societies. That health is now almost unrelated to measures of economic growth and yet closely related to income distribution suggests that priority must now be given to the satisfaction of social needs. It would be a mistake to respond to this situation by saying that we should forget about material progress and go solely for income distribution and an improvement in the social fabric of society. While there would be widespread agreement to the view that the condition of the social fabric of modern societies is often the most pressing limitation on the quality of life, it is important to recognise that much of what is valuable in the concept of civilisation rests at least loosely on material progress. The looseness of this attachment is shown by the way we regard the progress of civilisation as a historical rather than economic process – despite the obvious relation between the two. Our analysis of figure 3.1 suggests that it now has more to do with the qualitative change taking place over time than it does with the quantitative economic growth which – for instance – separates the standard of living in Greece or Ireland from that in the United States. While these countries are clearly all more civilised than they were a century ago, it is not clear that one is more civilised or has achieved more for human dignity among their populations than the others, despite the large differences in GNPpc between them. The improvement over time, combined with the lack of predominance of one developed country over another at a particular point, is highly concordant with the puzzle of figure 3.1.

If this is roughly right, it implies that we need to drop the crude identification of the quality of life with average level of material consumption and demote economic growth from its role as a societal goal. In its place we must operationalise values of human social and material emancipation, ensuring that narrower income differences extend dignity to all and so provide a material base conducive to the proper development of the social life of our societies.

Within the environmental limitations on resource use and the production of waste, we can still enjoy the products of scientific advance and technical innovation. In order to achieve those goals a new family of socioeconomic measures is needed. To draw attention to the important increases in material standards resulting from qualitative change we need – despite the formidable technical problems – properly quality-adjusted price indices. Perhaps it would also be possible to separate measures of qualitative improvements in goods and services from measures of resource use and waste production.

But how do we achieve a narrower income distribution and better social cohesion? The first step is for politicians and the public to recognise the importance of these issues. At the moment the management of the national economy is devoted almost exclusively to the pursuit of economic objectives. This must be changed. Policies on education, employment, industrial structure, taxation, the management of the business cycle, must all be assessed in terms of their impact on social justice and social divisions. Economic management must have the explicit aim of increasing social cohesion and the social quality of life.

Historical experience shows that political will is crucial. Rather than the necessary policy changes having to wait until the economy is 'right' and such social luxuries can be afforded, we saw in chapter 6 that, in wartime Britain, they became necessities. The redistribution of income, the guarantee of minimum standards for all, policies to ensure that the burden of war taxation did not fall disproportionately on the poor, the lowering of the social hierarchy, and plans for a massive expansion of the welfare state, all became urgently necessary as part of the effort to gain maximum co-operation in the war effort. Nor is this an isolated example. The World Bank's publication *The East Asian miracle* (World Bank 1993) has brief descriptions of the political pressures which led to a substantial narrowing of income differentials in all eight of the rapidly growing Asian economies (Japan, Republic of Korea, Taiwan, Singapore, Hong Kong, Thailand, Malaysia and Indonesia. China, which might have been a ninth, was outside their remit.) Again, rather than greater social equity appearing as a luxury that can only be afforded when countries had reached some illusory point where more pressing economic problems have been dealt with, it appears as a policy which, despite bringing substantial economic benefits (Birdsall *et al.* 1995), governments pursue only as a solution to political crises. In a chapter entitled 'An institutional basis for shared growth', the World Bank explains the move to greater equity in these Asian countries. It says that in each of them except Japan,

> new leaders faced an urgent need to establish their political viability before the economic take-off. The Republic of Korea was threatened by invasion from the North; Taiwan from China; and Thailand from Vietnam and Cambodia. In Indonesia, Malaysia, Singapore, and Thailand, leaders faced formidable communist threats. In addition, leaders in Indonesia, Korea and Taiwan, having taken power, needed to prove their ability to

govern. Leaders in Malaysia and Singapore had to contend with ethnic diversity and attendant questions of political representation. Even in Japan, where the competition was less immediate, leaders had to earn public confidence after the debacle of World War II. In all cases then, leaders desperately needed to answer a basic question: why should they lead and not others? Whatever strategy the leaders of these governments selected to answer the basic challenge of legitimacy, they included a *principle of shared growth*.

(World Bank 1993, p. 157)

The authors of the World Bank report describe the policies explicitly aimed at creating greater equality. They also point out that most of these policies did not involve direct income transfers from rich to poor but were aimed instead at overcoming obstacles and disadvantages to people's economic achievement. Among the approaches they used were land reform and land redistribution, universal education, increased employment opportunities, and intervention in the housing market to provide low-cost housing. It is clear however that what pushed them into these policies was – as it had been in Britain – war or the threat of it, the challenge of communist rivals, and resulting crises of legitimacy.

The traditional argument against equality is the frequently repeated suggestion that it involves sacrificing economic growth. We are told that a choice has to be made between equity and growth, and that smaller income differences would reduce incentives. However, there are now a number of empirical studies which show that, rather than having to choose between equity and growth, growth tends to be faster where there is more equity. The eight rapidly growing Asian economies covered by the World Bank report provide one example: they all narrowed their income distribution between 1960 and 1980 and Birdsall *et al.* have analysed some of the ways in which greater equity has assisted growth (Birdsall *et al.* 1995; World Bank 1993). A second example comes in a paper by Persson and Tabellini (1994) which provides two separate tests of the effect of income inequality on the growth rate of GDPpc. The first is a historical analysis going back from 1985 as far as data from a group of nine OECD countries allow. The units of observation are changes during each twenty-year period in each country. The second uses data for sixty-seven countries from 1950 (or 1960 where earlier data was unavailable) to 1985. Both test results show a robust relationship such that wider income differences are associated with slower growth. But, like Birdsall *et al.*, they were also able to show that the direction of causality was from equality to growth. Alesina and Perotti (1993) took data from some seventy developed and less developed countries and found that investment tended to be higher in countries with narrower income differences. They suggested that wider income differences reduced investment by contributing to political instability. Finally, Glyn found that among a group of sixteen OECD countries for which the World Bank had income distribution data, there was a clear tendency for more egalitarian countries to have bigger increases in labour productivity in the period 1979–90 (Glyn and Miliband 1994).

There are numerous ways in which greater equity is likely to benefit growth, including some which involve feedback effects creating virtuous circles. For instance, Birdsall emphasises how greater income equity and lower unemployment made families value education more highly and so stimulated economic growth. She says that by increasing the relative abundance of educated labour and eroding the scarcity value of the more highly educated, educational expansion and the simultaneous reduction in the inequality of educational opportunity reduced the inequality of income distribution. Feeding back to faster growth and lower income inequality, this further increased the supply of, and demand for, education. But even holding education constant, Birdsall found that greater income equity aided growth in these Asian countries. She suggested that it also increased family investment in forms of human capital other than education, and increased the domestic multiplier effect of increases in income initiated elsewhere in the economic system.

Inequality imposes numerous costs on the economy and society. As well as those we have discussed in the preceding chapters, there are other volumes that discuss evidence of a range of economic and social costs (Taylor 1990; Glyn and Miliband 1994). Most fundamentally, inequality turns a large proportion of the population from net contributors to a society's economic welfare into net burdens on it. There is no need to recap on the effects on health, children's emotional welfare, educational performance, accidents and crime which we have discussed in earlier chapters. With modern economic systems facing increasing international competition, few countries can afford to waste potentially valuable human resources by failing to make the necessary educational investments. By denying people the opportunity to experience themselves as valued members of society contributing to the economy, they have no choice but to add to the social security bill. But it is not merely these visible and calculable ways in which potential contributors are turned into welfare dependants, nor is it even the incalculable human costs of blighted lives, insecurity and frustration which relative poverty causes. Perhaps the most important effect on economic efficiency is the reduction of good-will and co-operation among the public at large. Employees who feel bitterness and antagonism towards their employer will be much less productive than people who are appreciated as members of a co-operative team and feel purposeful about their work. Some of the same processes are likely to operate throughout society, turning the pleasure of mutual co-operation into the destructive-ness and inefficiency of antagonism.

Increasingly we live in what might be called a 'cash and keys' society. Whenever we leave the confines of our own homes we face the world with the two perfect symbols of the nature of social relations on the street. Cash equips us to take part in transactions mediated by the market, while keys protect our private gains from each other's envy and greed. What adds to the social potency of these arrangements is that instead of being marginal to our lives, they are the organising principles of the most highly interdependent system of production and consumption that has ever existed. Although we are all wholly dependent on one another for our livelihoods, this interdependence is turned from being a social process into a process by which we fend for ourselves in an attempt to wrest a living from an asocial environment. Instead of being people with whom we have social bonds and share common interests, others become rivals, competitors for jobs, for houses, space, seats on the bus, parking places. And yet, as social beings, we cannot treat others in the arena of public life simply as part of the natural environment: instead processes of social comparison – favourable or unfavourable – mean everything is constantly monitored. We feel hurt, angry, belittled, annoyed and sometimes superior as the processes of social distinction and social exclusion thread their way between us. Add to this the major material inequalities and social injustices that exist in our society and we have a recipe which is hardly conducive to the most efficient and harmonious social order.

A study that beautifully illustrates the delicacy of the relationship between the market, poverty, social cohesion and health is Titmuss's *The gift relationship: from human blood to social policy* (1970) which compared the systems for collecting blood for transfusion in Britain and the USA. With the National Health Service, which made medical care free to all, there was in Britain no commercial market in blood. It was given by donors without any material rewards or inducements and made available freely to patients who needed transfusions. The National Blood Transfusion Service depended wholly on a form of public spiritedness which made people willing to donate blood through a non-commercial health service to unknown recipients. In contrast, during the later 1960s when the study was conducted, blood was collected in the USA through a number of different arrangements, but an increasing proportion was collected by profit-making blood banks which paid donors and sold it to hospitals for patients who had to pay for it. The differences in the way the two systems worked meant that blood was collected from very different sources in each society. In Britain it came from something close to a cross-section of society – except for a slight over-representation of higher-income groups and the policy of excluding older people and expectant and nursing mothers. In the USA, of those who sold their blood, it was found that 'the great majority are men, unskilled or semi-skilled workers or migrants on low earnings or unemployed' (Titmuss 1970, p. 126). Some of the commercial blood banks had arranged monopoly rights to collect blood from prisons and in some states prisoners were given a few days' remission for each pint they gave. 'Many commercial blood banks, often opening from 7.30 in the morning to midnight, are better placed to attract walk-in donors because their store fronts are located in ghetto areas. In 1966 voluntary and private hospitals bought 100,000 pints of skid row blood from New York City's 31 pay-for-blood stores (ibid., p. 127). (This was a little over 40 per cent of all the blood collected in New York.)

But the point is not primarily that this led to the collection of poor-quality blood supplies from people who had higher rates of hepatitis, venereal diseases, jaundice, drug addiction and alcoholism (the so-called 'ooze for booze' donors), and an interest in not declaring their condition. Nor is it that this led to a much higher death rate in the USA among patients receiving transfusions. The main point in the present context is that a non-commercial health service which provided patients with medical care and blood freely as they needed it, elicited a willingness among the public to make entirely voluntary donations of blood to unknown recipients on a scale large enough to meet the society's blood needs. (About one in thirty of the eligible population were donors.) On the same basis the National Health Service was also able to call on a fund of goodwill to provide a range of other systems of voluntary help and donations, ranging from the Hospital Car Service and voluntary workers in hospital to organ donations.

In many areas of life people are prepared to do voluntary work for charities and non-profit-making organisations. They may do very much the same tasks as people are paid to do elsewhere in the economy. But a commercial, profit-making organisation is – almost whatever its business – unable to call on voluntary help. However worthwhile the cause, to give one's labour voluntarily to a profit-making organisation is unacceptable: people would feel used and taken advantage of. It was interesting to note that when the public utilities – particularly water companies – were privatised in Britain during the 1980s and early 1990s, there was a clear loss of a co-operative public attitude to them. If water was provided on a profit-making basis, then people were much less willing to limit their consumption during droughts to help maintain water levels in reservoirs. Instead of using water sparingly as part of a voluntary willingness to conserve community supplies, it became the job of the company to sort their problems out and give people the service they paid for – whatever the difficulties. In almost all cases the privatisation of previously nationalised utilities led to a reduction of public tolerance: regardless of what happened to standards of services, there were substantial increases in the number of complaints they received.

What Titmuss emphasises in his study of blood donors is that systems that permit and elicit voluntary giving not only create opportunities for people to express and realise themselves through altruism and public spiritedness, but also create and strengthen some kind of cohesive moral community. It is worth remembering that what may seem remote issues to do with the formal structure and constitution of organisations can have a major impact on how they fit into society, whether or not they contribute to a sense of sharing, of common purpose and of social solidarity. The common provision of egalitarian systems of education, health care, transport, water and other basic services can no doubt make a contribution to a sense of belonging to a society.

While the example of blood donors provides a very neat example of at least one way in which social cohesion has a direct effect on health, Titmuss was also keen to point out that the voluntary system of blood donation was more efficient than the commercial one in every sense. It had lower social costs in terms of the people the blood came from; it had lower administrative costs; it was cheaper in economic terms; and it was safer for patients.

There can be no doubt that economic systems that destroy a spirit of social co-operation may incur very high additional costs as a result. Although an official report on the costs of crime avoided adding up the component estimates, they have been estimated elsewhere at 10 per cent of UK national income (Kelly 1993; Standing conference on crime prevention 1988). One of the fastest-growing areas of employment in the USA over the last decade has been additional security staff and janitors. But there are huge costs of crime prevention that do not come into any estimates. Indeed, the whole cost of running a monetary system, with accountants, cash machines, pricing, checkouts, wages staff, is all part of the administrative cost of running the modern interdependent productive system which does not rest on social co-operation. The lower the level of trust and co-operation, the more expensive it gets. How long will it be, for example, before filling stations have to install automatic barriers to prevent drivers leaving before they have paid for petrol?

Although Putnam contrasts his view of a well-developed 'civic community' with the 'a-moral familism' of a society in which public life is dominated by self-interest and cynicism, that conception came from Banfield's study of peasant society in southern Italy in the 1950s. Perhaps a more appropriate view of public life in a developed society with lower levels of social capital comes, not simply from the growth of problems associated with relative poverty, but from something closer to Rathbone's concept of a 'criminal society'. Just as Rose suggested that the overall distribution of a population's exposure to health risk factors moves up or down as a whole, the crime writer Julian Rathbone seems to have a similar view of levels of criminality reflecting a society's moral tone. He says:

We live in a criminal society. I mean a society that is structurally criminal. If we removed from our economy every trace of exploitation of the third world and actively worked in the opposite direction . . . if we wiped out all unnecessary pollution

... if we removed all traces of sexism and racism ... if we had a police force, a clergy, a judiciary, a parliament we could respect and trust ... if we wiped out all white collar crime in all its forms ... if we stopped selling weapons of destruction to homicidal maniacs ... if there was one single political party interested in structural justice rather than getting their bums onto [the government seats] ... if, if, if, then we might say our society is not structurally criminal.

(Rathbone 1995, p. 35)

The health effects of inequality have shown us how deeply people are affected by these structural features of our society. But even more important than the few extra years which greater equity would add to the average length of life is the improvement in the social quality of life which it would also give us. Not only is the cost of inequality a cost we incur for no economic benefit, but all the indications are that it imposes a substantial economic burden which reduces the competitiveness of the whole society.

It is clear that the psychosocial burden we have identified is now the most important limitation on the quality of life in modern societies. Instead of thinking in terms of economic growth and raising the material standard of living as the primary goal to which governments aspire, it is important that we take a more discriminating view of its benefits. To suggest that the links between income inequality and health operate primarily through psychosocial pathways, and that more egalitarian societies are more socially cohesive, will no doubt make some think that it is possible to skip the egalitarianism and go straight to attempts to make improvements in cohesion at the psychosocial level. When coping with the increasing range of social problems thrown up by the lack of cohesion and social justice, there is always a tendency to demand new services to deal with them. But, as we saw in chapter 2, this is an expensive and often ineffective response. Rather than relying on providing more special needs classes in schools, more prisons and police, more social workers and health services, more counsellors and therapists, we have to tackle at root some of the main causes of the problems with which they attempt to cope. Even if we could afford vast armies of counsellors and community development workers with a small team for every street, there is no reason to think that it is possible to separate the structural causes from their social symptoms. The important implication of the links which have been demonstrated in the preceding chapters is quite the other way round. At last we have a variable which is amenable to public policy and capable of improving the psychosocial well-being of the whole population. While politicians will no doubt shelter behind a set of reasons why they cannot make any substantial impact on income distribution, the evidence from the experience of Britain and a number of other countries is, once again, the other way round: income distribution is narrowed only when governments believe they cannot afford not to narrow it. However, as we get to know more about its social, economic and human effects, and people become increasingly aware of the costs of doing nothing, it seems likely that the political will be found.

Three points mentioned in chapter 2 are perhaps worth repeating as they provide some grounds for optimism. The first concerns the extraordinary increase in public awareness of health inequalities which has taken place over the last twenty years. Initially, when the subject of social class differences in death rates came up in conversation with doctors and others involved in healthcare, the first question was usually to ask which way round the differences were. Even among professionals concerned with health there was no recognition that standards of health were so much worse lower down the social scale. Since then, the relationship between poverty and poor health has become common knowledge and people are more likely to wonder if there is anything to be said about it which hasn't already been said. This transformation of public awareness has come about as a result of the repeat coverage by the media of a constant stream of research findings on numerous different aspects of the size and causes of the health differences.

The second reason for optimism concerns the response of politicians to the public attention given to the danger of hypothermia. The knowledge that old people may die during cold winters as a result of being unable to afford adequate heating resulted not only in headlines in the press drawing attention to this scandal whenever there was a cold winter. It also led politicians, who spent most of their time parading their desire for cuts in public expenditure as if it were a virility symbol, to take two steps: first, to vote in a special system of cold weather payments for pensioners and those on family income supplement; and second, to fight their own government in an attempt to forestall the addition of value added tax to fuel bills. In the end the government only won their support after agreeing to phase the tax in slowly while compensating the least well-off for the additional cost. If it was as widely recognised that hypothermia was just the tip of the iceberg, and that relative poverty and inequality accounted for many thousands of extra deaths a year, then perhaps politicians would feel obliged to bow to public opinion on these issues more often.

The third reason for optimism is that many of the results of greater inequality which we have discussed in this book do not affect the poor alone. Action does not depend simply on a sense of altruistic concern for the welfare of a minority. The majority cannot enjoy life oblivious to these problems: they affect the quality of life of all of us.

Bibliography

Action on Smoking and Health. *Her share of misfortune*. ASH, London. 1993.

Advisory Centre for Education. *Findings from the ACE investigations into exclusions*. ACE, London. 1993.

Alesina, A. and Perotti, R. *Income distribution, political instability, and investment*. NBER Working Paper 4486. National Bureau of Economic Research, Cambridge, Mass. 1993.

Andrews, E. Japanese gangs learn to say sorry. *The Guardian*, 7 September 1995.

Antonovsky, A. Can attitudes contribute to health? *Advances* 8: 33–49. 1992.

Aoki, M. and Dore, R.P. (eds) *The Japanese firm: sources of competitive strength*. Oxford University Press, Oxford. 1994.

Arber, S. Social class, non-employment, and chronic illness: continuing the inequalities in the health debate. *British Medical Journal*, 294: 1069–73. 1987.

Atkinson, A.B. and Micklewright, J. *The distribution of income in Eastern Europe*. Working paper 72, Welfare State Programme, LSE, London. 1992a.

Atkinson, A.B. and Micklewright, J. *Economic transformation in Eastern Europe and the distribution of income*. Cambridge, Cambridge University Press. 1992b.

Backlund, E., Sorlie, P.D. and Johnson, N.J. The shape of the relationship between income and mortality in the United States: evidence from the National Longitudinal Mortality Study. *Annals of Epidemiology* 6: 12–20. 1996.

Balkwell, J. Ethnic inequality and the rate of homicide. *Social Forces* 69: 53–70. 1990.

Banfield, E.C. *The moral basis of a backward society*. Free Press, Glencoe, Ill. 1958.

Bartley, M. Unemployment and ill-health: understanding the relationship. *Journal of Epidemiology and Community Health* 48 (4): 333–7. 1994.

Bartley, M. and Plewis, I. Relationship between social mobility and illness in England and Wales 1971–91. *Journal of Health and Social Behaviour.* Forthcoming 1996.

Bayley, D.H. *Forces of order: police behavior in Japan and the United States.* University of California Press, Berkeley. 1976.

Beckerman, W. *Small is stupid: blowing the whistle on the Greens.* Duckworth, London. 1995.

Bem, D. Self perception theory. In: *Advances in experimental social psychology*, Vol. 6. Edited by L. Berkowitz. Academic Press, NY. 1972.

Ben Shlomo, Y., White, I.R. and Marmot, M. Does the variation in the socioeconomic characteristics of an area affect mortality? *British Medical Journal* 1996; 312: 1013–14.

Bennathan, M. and Smith, H. The state of services for children in London. *Young Minds Newsletter* 8: 10–12. 1991.

Bennet, G. British floods 1968: controlled survey of effects on health of local community disaster. *British Medical Journal* 3: 454–8. 1970.

Berkman, L.F. The role of social relations in health promotion. *Psychosomatic Research* 57: 245–54. 1995.

Berkman, L.F. and Syme, S.L. Social networks, host resistance and mortality: a nine year follow up study of Alameda County residents. *American Journal of Epidemiology.* 109: 186. 1979.

Birdsall, N., Ross, D. and Sabot, R. Inequality and growth reconsidered – lessons from East-Asia. *World Bank Economic Review* 9 (3): 477–508. 1995.

Blane, D., Davey Smith, G. and Bartley, M. Social selection: what does it contribute to social class differences in health? *Sociology of Health and Illness*; 15: 1–15. 1993.

Blaus, J. and Blaus, P. The costs of inequality: metropolitan structure and violent crime. *American Sociological Review* 47: 121. 1982.

Blaxter, M. *Health and Lifestyles.* Routledge, London. 1990.

Bourdieu, P. *Distinction: a social critique of the judgement of taste.* Routledge, London. 1984.

Braithwaite, J. *Inequality, crime and public policy.* Routledge, London. 1979.

Braithwaite, J. *Crime, shame and reintegration.* Cambridge University Press, Cambridge. 1989.

Braithwaite, J. and Braithwaite, V. The effect of income inequality and social democracy on homicide. *British Journal of Criminology* 20 (1): 45–53. 1980.

Broadhead, W.E., Kaplan, B.H., James, S.A., *et al.* The epidemiologic evidence for a relationship between social support and health. *American Journal of Epidemiology* 117: 521–37. 1983.

Brown, G.W. Social class, psychiatric disorder of mother, and accidents to children. *Lancet* 1: 378. 1978.

Bruhn, J.G. and Wolf, S. *The Roseto Story.* University of Oklahoma Press, Norman. 1979.

Brunner, E. The social and biological basis of cardiovascular disease in office workers. In: *Health and Social Organisation.* Edited by Brunner, E., Blane, D. and Wilkinson, R.G. Routledge, London. 1996.

Building Societies Yearbook 1993/4. As quoted in: *Moneywise*, p. 36, October 1993.

Bunker, J.P., Frazier, H.S. and Mosteller, F. Improving health: measuring effects of medical care. *Millbank Quarterly* 72 (2): 225–58. 1994.

Burgoyne, J. Unemployment and married life. *Unemployment Bulletin* 18: 7–10. 1985.

Burnet, F.M. and White, D.O. *The natural history of infectious disease*. 4th edn. Cambridge University Press, Cambridge. 1972.

Cameron, D. and Jones, I.G. An epidemiological and sociological analysis of the use of alcohol, tobacco and other drugs of solace. *Community Medicine* 7: 18–29. 1985.

Champoux, M., Coe, C.L., Shanberg, S., Kuhn, C. and Soumi, S.J. Hormonal effects of early rearing conditions in the infant rhesus monkey. *American Journal of Primatology* 19: 111–17. 1989.

Clifford, W. *Crime control in Japan*. Lexington Books, Lexington, Mass. 1976.

Cobb, S. and Kasl, S.C. *Termination: the consequences of job loss*. Cincinnati: Department of Health, Education and Welfare – US National Institutes for Occupational Safety and Health, publication no. 77–224, US NIOSH. 1977.

Cohen, S., Tyrrell, D.A.J. and Smith, A.P. Psychological stress and susceptibility to the common cold. *New England Journal of Medicine* 325: 606–12. 1991.

Conduit, E.H. If A–B does not predict heart disease, why bother with it? A clinician's view. *British Journal of Medical Psychology*. 65: 289–96. 1992.

Creighton, S.J. *Child abuse trends in England and Wales 1988–90 and an overview from 1973–1990*. NSPCC, London. 1992.

Crutchfield, R. Labor stratification and violent crime. *Social Forces* 68: 589–612. 1989.

Currie, E. *Confronting crime*. Pantheon, NY. 1985.

Daley, H.E. and Cobb, J.B. *For the Common Good*. Green Print, London. 1990.

Davey Smith, G., Shipley, M.J. and Rose, G. Magnitude and causes of socioeconomic differentials in mortality: further evidence from the Whitehall Study. *Journal of Epidemiology and Community Health* 44: 265–70. 1990.

Davey Smith, G., Neaton, J.D. and Stamler, J. Socioeconomic differentials in mortality risk among men screened for the Multiple Risk Factor Intervention Trial. White men. *American Journal of Public Health* 1996. 86: 486–96.

Deci, E.L. Effects of externally mediated rewards on intrinsic motivation. *Journal of Personality and Social Psychology* 18: 105–15. 1971.

DeMause, L. (ed.) *The History of Childhood*. Condor, London. 1974.

Department of Health. *On the state of the public health. Annual report of the chief medical officer 1990*. HMSO, London. 1991.

Department of Health. *Health Survey for England 1991*. HMSO, London. 1993.

Department of Social Security. *Households below average income 1979–1990/1*. HMSO, London. 1993.

Dore, R. *British factory – Japanese factory. The origins of national diversity in industrial relations*. University of California Press, Berkeley. 1973.

Dore, R. Seminar, 20 June, International Centre for Health and Society, University College London, and personal communication. 1995.

Dore, R. The limits of discontinuity. Unpublished paper 1996.

Dunn, J. and Plomin, R. Why are siblings so different? The significance of differences in sibling experiences within the family. *Family Process* 10: 271–83. 1991.

Durkheim, E. *Suicide*. Edited by G. Simpson. Routledge, London. 1952.

Egolf, B., Lasker, J., Wolf, S. and Potvin, L. The Roseto effect: a 50-year comparison of mortality rates. *American Journal of Public Health* 82: 1089–92. 1992.

Eyer, J. Capitalism, health, and illness. In: *Issues in the political economy of health care*. Edited by J.B. McKinlay, Tavistock, NY. 1984.

Ferri, E. *Growing up in a one-parent family*. National Foundation for Educational Research. Slough. 1976.

Ferri, E. and Robinson, H. *Coping alone*. National Foundation for Educational Research. Slough. 1976.

Ferri. *Omicidio-suicidio*. 4th edn. Turin. 1895.

Ferrie, J.E., Shipley, M.J., Marmot, M.G., Stansfield, S. and Davey Smith, G. Health effects of anticipation of job change and non-employment: longitudinal data from the Whitehall II study. *British Medical Journal* 311: 1264–9. 1995.

Firth, R. *The Economics of the New Zealand Maori*. R.E. Owen, Wellington, NZ. 1959.

Flegg, A. Inequality of income, illiteracy, and medical care as determinants of infant mortality in developing countries. *Population Studies* 36: 441–58. 1982.

Fox, J., Goldblatt, P. and Jones, D. Social class mortality differentials: artefact, selection or life circumstances? *Journal of Epidemiology and Community Health* 39: 1–8. 1985.

Gallerani, M., Manfredini, R. and Caracciolo, S., Scapoli, C., Molinari, S. and Fersini, C. Serum cholesterol concentrations in parasuicide. *British Medical Journal* 310: 1632–6. 1995.

Gellner, E. *The psychoanalytic movement: the cunning of unreason*. 2nd edn. Fontana, London. 1993.

Glyn, A. and Miliband, D. Introduction. In: *Paying for inequality: the costs of social injustice*. Edited. by A. Glyn and D. Miliband. Rivers Oram Press, London. 1994.

Goldblatt, P. Mortality and alternative social classifications. In: *Mortality and Social Organisation: Longitudinal Study 1971–81*. Series LS 6. Edited by P. Goldblatt. HMSO, London. 1990.

Goldsmith, M.M. *Private vices, public benefits*. Cambridge University Press, Cambridge. 1985.

Goodall, J. *The chimpanzees of Gombe: patterns of behavior*. Harvard University Press, Cambridge, Mass. 1986.

Goody, J. *Technology, tradition and the state in Africa*. Oxford University Press, Oxford. 1971.

Gorbachev, M. 'The way ahead . . . more democracy and openness', *The Guardian*. Monday 2 February 1987.

Gorman, T. and Fernandes, C. *Reading in recession*. National Foundation for Educational Research, Slough. 1992.

Greater Glasgow Health Board. *The annual report of the Director of Public Health 1991/2*. Greater Glasgow Health Board, Glasgow. 1993.

Gross, J.T. A note on the nature of Soviet totalitarianism. *Soviet Studies* 34: 367–76. 1982.

Grossman, M. *Demand for health: a theoretical and empirical investigation*. NBER, New York. 1972.

Haan, M., Kaplan, G.A. and Camacho, T. Poverty and health: prospective evidence from the Alameda County Study. *American Journal of Epidemiology* 125: 989–98. 1987.

Hajdu, P., McKee, M. and Bojan, F. Changes in premature mortality differentials by marital status in Hungary and England and Wales. *European Journal of Public Health* 5: 529–64. 1995.

Hayakawa, K., Shimizu, T., Ohba, Y., Tomioka, S., Takahasi, S. and Amano, K. Intrapair differences of physical aging and longevity in identical twins. *Acta Genetica Med. Gemellol* 41: 177–85. 1992a.

Hayakawa, K., Shimizu, T., Ohba, Y. and Tomioka, S. Risk factors for cognitive ageing in adult twins. *Acta Genetica Med. Gemellol* 41; 187–95. 1992b.

Helsing, K.J. and Szklo, M. Mortality after bereavement *American Journal of Epidemiology* 114: 41–52. 1981.

Hertzman, C. *Environment and Health in Central and Eastern Europe*. World Bank, Washington DC. 1995.

Hewlett, S.A. *Child neglect in rich nations*. UNICEF, New York. 1993.

Hills, J. *The future of welfare*. Joseph Rowntree Foundation, York. 1994.

Hills, J. *Inquiry into income and wealth*. Volume 2. Joseph Rowntree Foundation, York. 1995.

Himsworth, H. Epidemiology, genetics and sociology. *Journal of Biosocial Science* 16: 159–76. 1984.

House, J.S., Landis, K.R. and Umberson, D. Social relationships and health. *Science* 241: 540–5. 1988.

Illsley, R. Social class selection and class differences in relation to stillbirths and infant deaths. *British Medical Journal* 2: 1520–4. 1955.

Ineichen, B. *Homes and health: how housing and health interact*. Spon, London. 1993.

Institute for the Study of Drug Dependence. *National Audit of Drug Misuse in Britain 1994*. ISDD, London. 1994.

Institute for the Study of Drug Dependence. *National Audit of Drug Misuse in Britain 1992*. ISDD, London. 1992.

Iversen, L. and Klausen, H. *The closure of the Nordhavn shipyard*. Copenhagen: Institute of Social Medicine. Kobenhavns Universitet Publikation 13 FADL. 1981.

Jackson, T. and Marks, N. UK *Index of sustainable economic welfare*. Stockholm Environment Institute in cooperation with the New Economic Foundation. Stockholm, 1994.

James, O. *Juvenile violence in a winner–loser culture*. Free Association Books, London. 1995.

Johnson, J.V. and Hall, E.M. Job strain, work place social support, and cardiovascular disease: a cross-sectional study of a random sample of the Swedish working population. *American Journal of Public Health* 78: 1336–42. 1988.

Jones, A.M. *A microeconometric analysis of smoking in the UK Health and Lifestyle Survey*. Discussion paper 139, Centre for Health Economics, York. 1995.

Joseph Rowntree Foundation, *Social Policy Research Findings*. No. 37, York. May 1993.

Kaplan, G.A., Pamuk, E., Lynch, J.W., Cohen, R.D. and Balfour, J.L. Income inequality and mortality in the United States. *British Medical Journal* 1996; 312: 999–1003.

Kaplan, J.R., Shively, C.A. and Fontenot, M.B. *et al*. Demonstration of an association among dietary-cholesterol, central serotonergic activity, and social behaviour in monkeys. *Psychosomatic Medicine* 56: 479–84. 1994.

Karasek, R. and Theorell, T. *Healthy work: stress, productivity and the reconstruction of working life*. Basic Books, NY. 1990.

Karasek, R.A., Theorell, T., Schwartz, J., Schnall, P., Pieper, C. and Michela, J. Job characteristics in relation to the prevalence of myocardial infarction in the US HES and HANES. *American Journal of Public Health* 78: 910–18. 1988.

Kehrer, B.H. and Wolin, C.M. Impact of income maintenance on low birth weight: Evidence from the Gary experiment. *Journal of Human Resources* 14: 435–62. 1979.

Kelleher, C., Cooper, J. and Sadlier, D. ABO blood group and social class: a prospective study in a regional blood bank. *Journal of Epidemiology and Community Health* 44: 59–61. 1990.

Kelly, R. The invisible hand behind the inexorable increase in the rate of crime. *The Guardian*, 30 August, 1993.

Kennedy, B.P. and Kawachi, I. and Prothrow-Stith, D. Income distribution and mortality: Cross sectional ecological study of the Robin Hood Index in the United States. *British Medical Journal* 1996; 312: 1004–7.

Kennedy, S., Kiecolt-Glaser, J.K. and Glaser, R. Immunological consequences of acute and chronic stressors: mediating role of interpersonal relationships. *British Journal of Medical Psychology* 61: 77–85. 1988.

Kleinke, C.L. *Self-perception: the psychology of personal awareness*. W.H. Freeman, San Francisco. 1978.

Kochanek, K.D., Maurer, J.D., Rosenberg, M.S. and Rosenberg, H.M. Why did black life expectancy decline from 1984 through 1989 in the United States? *American Journal of Public Health* 84: 938–44. 1994.

Koskinen, S. Time trends in cause specific mortality by occupational class in England and Wales. In: *Proceedings of IUSSP conference held in Florence, June 1985*. Florence 1988.

Kunst, A.E. and Mackenbach, J.P. The size of mortality differences associated with educational level in nine industrialized countries. *American Journal of Public Health* 84: 932–7. 1994.

Kunst, A.E. and Mackenbach, J. International comparisons of socio-economic inequalities in mortality. *Social Science and Medicine.* Forthcoming 1996.

Lake, M. Surveying all the factors. *Language and Learning.* June No. 6. 1991.

Lambert, R. *Nutrition in Britain 1950–60.* Codicote Press, Welwyn. 1964.

Leclerc, A. Differential mortality by cause of death: comparisons between selected European countries. In: *Health inequalities in European countries.* Edited by A.J. Fox. Gower, Aldershot. 1989.

Leclerc, A., Lert, F. and Fabien, C. Differential mortality: some comparisons between England and Wales, Finland and France, based on inequality measures. *International Journal of Epidemiology* 19: 1001–10. 1990.

Le Grand, J. Inequalities in health: some international comparisons. *European Economic Review* 31: 182–91. 1987.

Leon, D.A. and Wilkinson, R.G. Inequalities in prognosis: socio-economic differences in cancer and heart disease survival. In: *Health inequalities in European countries.* Edited by A.J. Fox. Gower, Aldershot. 1989.

Leon, D.A., Vagero, D. and Otterblad Olausson, P. Social class differences in infant mortality in Sweden: a comparison with England and Wales. *British Medical Journal* 305: 687–91. 1992.

Lindberg, G., Rastam, L., Gullberg, B. and Eklund, G.A. Low serum cholesterol concentration and short-term mortality from injuries in men and women. *British Medical Journal* 305: 277–9. 1992.

London Borough of Croydon. *Reading competence at age 7.* Education Department, London Borough of Croydon. 1992.

Lowry, S. *Housing and health.* British Medical Journal Publishing, London. 1991.

Lundberg, O. Childhood living conditions, health status, and social mobility: a contribution to the health selection debate. *European Sociological Review* 7: 149–62. 1991.

Lundberg, O. The impact of childhood living conditions on illness and mortality in adulthood. *Social Science and Medicine* 36: 1047–52. 1993.

Lundberg, O. and Nystron Peck, M. Sense of coherence, social structure and health. *European Journal of Public Health*; 4: 252–7. 1994.

McCarron, P.G., Davey Smith, G. and Womersley, J.J. Deprivation and mortality in Glasgow from 1980 to 1992. *British Medical Journal* 309: 1481–2. 1994.

McCord, C. and Freeman, H.P. Excess mortality in Harlem. *New England Journal of Medicine* 322: 173–7. 1990.

McGowan, P. Lloyd's financial disaster 'has cost more than 30 lives'. *Evening Standard,* 18 February, 1994.

McIsaac, S. and Wilkinson, R.G. Cause of death, income distribution and problems of response rates. Luxembourg Income Study Working Paper 136. 1995 (EJPH 1996 forthcoming).

McKendrick, N., Brewer, J. and Plumb, J.H. *The birth of a consumer society: the commercialization of eighteenth-century England.* Europa Publications, London. 1982.

McKeown, T., Record, R.G. and Turner, R.D. An interpretation of the decline in mortality in England and Wales during the twentieth century. *Population Studies* 29: 391–422. 1975.

McLanahan, S. Family structure and the reproduction of poverty. *American Journal of Sociology* 90: 873–901. 1985.

McLoone, P. and Boddy, F.A. Deprivation and mortality in Scotland: 1981 and 1991. *British Medical Journal* 309: 1465–70. 1994.

Mackenbach, J.P., Bouvier-Colle, M.H. and Jougla, E. 'Avoidable' mortality and health services: a review of aggregate data studies. *Journal of Epidemiology and Community Health* 44: 106–11. 1990.

Mandeville, B. *The fable of the bees: or, private vices, publick benefits.* Penguin, Harmondsworth. 1970.

Marmot, M.G. Social inequalities in mortality: the social environment. In: *Class and health: research and longitudinal data.* Edited by R.G. Wilkinson. Tavistock, London. 1986.

Marmot, M.G., Davey Smith, G. Why are the Japanese living longer? *British Medical Journal* 299: 1547–51. 1989.

Marmot, M.G., Adelstein, A., Robinson, N. and Rose, G. Changing social class distribution of heart disease. *British Medical Journal* ii: 1109–12. 1978a.

Marmot, M.G., Rose, G., Shipley, M. and Hamilton, P.J.S. Employment grade and coronary heart disease in British civil servants. *Journal of Epidemiology and Community Health* 32: 244–9. 1978b.

Marmot, M.G., Shipley, M.J. and Rose, G. Inequalities in death – specific explanations of a general pattern. *Lancet* 1 (8384): 1003–6. 1984.

Marmot, M.G., Davey Smith, G., Stansfield, S., Patel, C., North, F. and Head, J. Health inequalities among British civil servants: the Whitehall II study *Lancet* 337: 1387–93. 1991.

Marsh, A. and McKay, S. *Poor Smokers.* Policy Studies Institute, London. 1994.

Marshall, L. Sharing, talking and giving: relief of social tensions among the !Kung Bushmen. *Africa* 31: 231–49. 1961.

Martini, C.J., Allan, G.H. and Davidson, J. Health indexes sensitive to medical care variation. *International Journal of Health Services* 7: 293–309. 1977.

Mascie-Taylor, C.G.N. *Biosocial aspects of social class.* Oxford University Press, Oxford. 1990.

Mattiasson, I., Lindgarde, F., Nilsson, J.A. and Theorell, T. Threat of unemployment and cardiovascular risk factors: longitudinal study of quality of sleep and serum cholesterol concentrations in men threatened with redundancy. *British Medical Journal* 301: 461–6. 1990.

Meaney, M.J., Aitken, D.H., van Berkel, C., Bhatnagar, S. and Sapolsky, R.M. Effect of neonatal handling on age-related impairments associated with the hippocampus. *Science* 239: 766–8. 1988.

Messner, S.F. Societal development, social equality and homicide. *Social Forces* 61. 1982.

Milward, A.S. *The economic effects of the two world wars.* Macmillan, London. 1984.

Mischel, W. *Introduction to personality: a new look.* (4th edn) Holt, NY. 1986.

Moller, S.E. Serotonin, carbohydrates, and atypical depression. *Pharmacology and Toxicology* 71: 61–71. 1992.

Montgomery, S.M. and Bartley, M.J. The association between slow growth in childhood and family conflict. Forthcoming. 1996.

Montgomery, S.M., Bartley, M.J., Cook, D.G. and Wadsworth, M.E.J. Health and social precursors of unemployment in young men. *Journal of Epidemiology and Community Health* 50. 1996.

Morris, J., Blane, D. and White, I.R. Levels of mortality, education and social conditions in the 107 LEAs of England. *Journal of Epidemiology and Community Health* 50: 15–17. 1996.

Multiple Risk Factor Intervention Trial Group. The Multiple Intervention Risk Factor Intervention Trial – risk factor changes and mortality results. *Journal of the American Medical Association* 248: 1465–76. 1982.

Nash, M. *Primitive and peasant economic systems*. Chandler Publishing Co., San Francisco 1966.

Nelson, R.A., Tanguay, T.L. and Patterson, C.D. A quality-adjusted price index for personal computers. *Journal of Business and Economic Statistics* 12: 23–31. 1994.

Nordhaus, W.D. Do real output and real wage measures capture reality? The history of lighting suggests not. NBER Working Paper and Cowles Foundation for Research in Economics at Yale, Discussion Paper 1078. 1994.

Nystrom Peck, A.M. Childhood environment, intergenerational mobility, and adult health – evidence from Swedish data. *Journal of Epidemiology and Community Health* 46: 71–4. 1992.

Nystrom Peck, M. and Lundberg, O. Short stature as an effect of economic and social conditions in childhood. *Social Science and Medicine* 41: 733–8. 1995.

O'Donnell, O. and Propper, C. *Equity and the distribution of National Health Service Resources*. Welfare State Programme Paper No. 45, London School of Economics, London. 1989.

OPCS. *Occupational Mortality: The Registrar General's decennial supplement for England and Wales 1970–2*. Series DS No.1. HMSO, London. 1978.

OPCS. *Mortality Statistics*. HMSO, London. 1991.

Pamuk, E. Social class inequality in mortality from 1921 to 1972 in England and Wales. *Population Studies* 39: 17–31. 1985.

Parker, H., Bakx, K. and Newcombe, R. *Living with heroin*. Open University Press, Milton Keynes. 1988.

Patel, C. and Marmot, M.G. Stress management, blood pressure and quality of life. *Journal of Hypertension* 5: S21–8. 1987.

Pavin, M. Economic determinants of political unrest: an economic approach. *Journal of Conflict Resolution* 17: 271–96. 1973.

Persson, T. and Tabellini, G. Is inequality harmful for growth? Theory and evidence. *American Economic Review* 84 (3): 600–21. 1994.

Phillimore, P., Beattie, A. and Townsend, P. The widening gap. Inequality of health in northern England, 1981–1991. *British Medical Journal* 308: 1125–8. 1994.

Platt, S. and Kreitman, N. Trends in parasuicide and unemployment among men in Edinburgh, 1968–82. *British Medical Journal* 289: 1029–32. 1984.

Plomin, R. and Daniels, D. Why are children in the same family so different from one another? *Behavioral and Brain Sciences* 10: 1–60. 1987.

Power, C., Manor, O., Fox, A.J. and Fogelman, K. Health in childhood and social inequalities in young adults. *Journal of the Royal Statistical Society* (series A) 153: 17–28. 1990.

Power, C., Manor, O. and Fox, J. *Health and class: the early years.* Chapman and Hall, London. 1991.

Power, C. and Manor, O. Asthma, enuresis, and chronic illness – long term impact on height. *Archives of Diseases in Childhood* 73 (4): 298–304. 1995.

Power, M. *The egalitarians – human and chimpanzee. An anthropological view of social organization.* Cambridge University Press, Cambridge. 1991.

Preston, S.H. The changing relation between mortality and level of economic development. *Population Studies* 29: 231–48. 1975.

Putnam, R.D., Tuning in, tuning out: the strange disappearance of social capital in America. *Political Science and Politics.* December: 664–83. 1995.

Putnam, R.D., Leonardi, R. and Nanetti, R.Y. *Making democracy work: civic traditions in modern Italy.* Princeton University Press, Princeton, NJ. 1993.

Radcliffe-Brown, A.R. *The Anderman Islanders.* Free Press, Glencoe, Ill. 1948.

Rathbone, J. Character assassination. *New Statesman and Society.* 15 December 1995.

Redpath, B. Family Expenditure Survey: a second study of differential response, comparing census characteristics of FES respondents and non-respondents. *Statistical News* 72: 13–16. 1986.

Rodgers, G.B. Income and inequality as determinants of mortality: an international cross-section analysis. *Population Studies* 33: 343–51. 1979.

Rose, G. Strategy of prevention: lessons from cardiovascular disease. *British Medical Journal* 282: 1847–51. 1981.

Rose, G. Sick individuals and sick populations. *International Journal of Epidemiology* 14: 32–8. 1985.

Rose, G. *The strategy of preventive medicine.* Oxford University Press, Oxford. 1992.

Rosengren, A., Orth-Gomer, K., Wedel, H. and Wilhelmsen, L. Stressful life events, social support, and mortality in men born in 1933. *British Medical Journal* 307: 1102–5. 1993.

Ross, C.E. and Huber, J. Hardship and depression. *Journal of Health and Social Behaviour* 26: 312–27. 1985.

Ross, L. The intuitive psychologist and his shortcomings: distortions in the attribution process. In: *Cognitive theories in social psychology.* Edited by L. Berkowitz. Academic Press, NY. 1978.

Sahlins, M. *Stone Age Economics.* Tavistock, London. 1974.

Sapolsky, R.M. Poverty's remains. *The Sciences* 31: 8–10. New York. 1991.

Sapolsky, R.M. *Stress, the aging brain, and mechanisms of neuron death.* MIT Press, Cambridge, Mass. 1992.

Sapolsky, R.M. Endocrinology alfresco: psychoendocrine studies of wild baboons. *Recent Progress in Hormone Research* 48: 437–68. 1993.

Sapolsky, R.M. *Why zebras don't get ulcers. A guide to stress, stress-related disease and coping.* W.H. Freeman, New York. 1994.

Saunders, P. *Aiming high: meritocracy in Britain.* Institute of Economic Affairs, London. 1996.

Sawyer, M. *Income distribution in OECD countries.* OECD Economic Outlook; Occasional Studies: 3–36. 1976.

Schapera, I. *The Khoisan peoples of South Africa.* Routledge, London. 1930.

Schwartz, R.D. and Orleans, S. On legal sanctions. *University of Chicago Law Review*, 34: 274–300. 1967.

Schwartz, S. The fallacy of the ecological fallacy: the potential misuse of a concept and the consequences. *American Journal of Public Health* 84: 819–24. 1994.

Schweinhart, L.J. and Weikart, D.P. Success by empowerment: The High/Scope Perry Preschool Study through age 27. *Young Children* 49: 54–8. 1993.

Sen, A. Public action and the quality of life in developing countries. *Oxford Bulletin of Economics and Statistics* 43: 287–319. 1981.

Sennett, R. and Cobb, J. *The Hidden Injuries of Class.* Knopf, NY. 1973.

Shannon, T. and Morgan, C. *The invisible crying tree.* Doubleday, London. 1996.

Siegal, D. Errors in output deflators revisited: unit values and the producer price index. *Economic Inquiry* 32: 11–32. 1994.

Siegrist, J., Peter, R., Junge, A., Cremer, P. and Seidel, D. Low status control, high effort at work and ischaemic heart disease: prospective evidence from blue-collar men. *Social Science and Medicine* 31: 1127–34. 1990.

Simecka, M. *The restoration of order: the normalisation of Czechoslovakia.* Verso, London. 1984.

Slater, C.H., Lorimor, R.J. and Lairson, D.R. The independent contributions of socioeconomic status and health practices to health status. *Preventive Medicine* 14: 372–78. 1985.

Smith, D. Despairing middle class fearful about the future. *Sunday Times*, 26 June 1994.

Stabler, B. and Underwood, L.E. (eds) *Slow grows the child: psychosocial aspects of growth delay.* Lawrence Erlbaum, Hillsdale, New Jersey. 1986.

Standing conference on crime prevention. Working Group on the costs of crime. Home Office. *Report of the working group on the costs of crime.* Home Office, London. 1988.

Statistics Bureau, Japan. *Japan Statistical Yearbook.* Statistics Bureau, Management and Coordination Agency. 1990.

Steckel, R.H. Height and per capita income. *Historical Methods* 16: 1–7. 1983.

Steckel, R.H. Heights and health in the United States. In: *Stature, living standards and economic development*. Edited by J. Komlos. University of Chicago Press, Chicago. 1994.

Susser, M. The logic in ecological: I. The logic of analysis. *American Journal of Public Health* 84: 825–9. 1994.

Sweeting, H. and West, P. Family life and health in adolescence: a role for culture in health inequalities? *Social Science and Medicine* 40: 163–75. 1995.

Syme, S.L. To prevent disease: the need for a new approach. In: *Health and social organization*. Edited by D. Blane, E. Brunner and R.G. Wilkinson. Routledge, London. 1996.

Szreter, S. The importance of social intervention in Britain's mortality decline c. 1850–1914: a reinterpretation of the role of public health. *Social History of Medicine* 1: 1–37. 1988.

Tarkowska, E. and Tarkowski, J. Social disintegration in Poland: civil society or amoral familism? *Telos* 89: 103–9. 1991.

Taylor, I. (ed.) *The social effects of free market policies*. Harvester Wheatsheaf, Hertfordshire. 1990.

Taylor, J.C., Norman, C.L., Griffiths, J.M., Anderson, H.R. and Ramsey, J.D. *Trends in deaths associated with abuse of volatile substances 1971–1991*. Dept. of Public Health Sciences and the Toxicology Unit, St George's Hospital Medical School, London. 1993.

Tennant, C.C., Palmer, K.J., Langgeluddecke, P.M., Jones, M.P. and Nelson, G. Life event stress and myocardial reinfarction: a prospective study. *European Heart Journal* 15: 472–8. 1994.

Timio, M., Verdecchia, P., Venanzi, S., Gentili, S., Ronconi, M., Francucci, B., Montanari, M. and Bichisao, E. Age and blood pressure changes: a 20-year follow up study in nuns in a secluded order. *Hypertension* 12: 457–61. 1988.

Titmuss, R.M. War and social policy In: *Essays on the welfare state*. Edited by R.M. Titmuss. Unwin, London. 1958.

Titmuss, R.M. *The gift relationship: from human blood to social policy*. Allen & Unwin, London. 1970.

Townsend, P. *Poverty in the United Kingdom*. Penguin, Harmondsworth. 1979.

Townsend P., Phillimore P. and Beattie, A. *Health and deprivation: inequality and the north*. Croom Helm, London. 1988.

Ullah, P. The association between income, financial strain and psychological well-being among unemployed youths. *Journal of Occupational Psychology* 63: 317–30. 1990.

UNICEF. *The Progress of Nations 1993*. UNICEF, New York. 1993.

Uno, H., Tarara, R., Else, J.G., Suleman, M.A. and Sapolsky, R.M. Hippocampal damage associated with prolonged fatal stress in primates. *Journal of Neuroscience* 9: 1705–11. 1989.

Vagero, D. and Lundberg, O. Health inequalities in Britain and Sweden. *Lancet* 2: 35–6. 1989.

van Doorslaer, E., Wagstaff, A., Bleichrodt, H., *et al*. Socioeconomic inequalities in health: some international comparisons. *Journal of Health Economics* 1996.

Vogel, E.F. From friendship to comradeship: the change in personal relations in communist China. *China Quarterly* 21: 46–70. 1965.

Wadsworth, M.E.J. Early stress and associations with adult health, behaviour and parenting. In: *Stress and disability in childhood*. Edited by R.N. Butler and B.D. Corner. Wright, Bristol. 1984.

Wadsworth, M.E.J. Serious illness in childhood and its association with later-life achievement. In: *Class and health: research and longitudinal data*. Edited by R.G. Wilkinson. Tavistock, London. 1986.

Wadsworth, M., Maclean M., Kuh, D. and Rodgers, B. Children of divorced and separated parents: summary and review of findings from a long-term follow-up study in the UK. *Family Practice* 7: 104–9. 1990.

Waldmann, R.J. Income distribution and infant mortality. *Quarterly Journal of Economics* 107: 1283–302. 1992.

Waldron, I., Nowotarski, M., Freimer, M., Henry, J.P., Post, N. and Witten, C. Cross-cultural variation in blood pressure: a quantitative analysis of the relationships of blood pressure to cultural characteristics, salt consumption and body weight. *Social Science and Medicine* 16: 419–30. 1982.

Wardle, J. Cholesterol and psychological well-being. *Journal of Psychosomatic Research* 39: 549–62. 1995.

Watson, P. Explaining rising mortality among men in Eastern Europe. *Social Science and Medicine* 41: 923–34. 1995.

Wennemo, I. Infant mortality, public policy and inequality – a comparison of 18 industrialised countries 1950–85. *Sociology of Health and Illness* 15: 429–46. 1993.

Wheaton, B. The sociogenesis of psychological disorder: an attributional theory. *Journal of Health and Social Behaviour* 21: 100–23. 1980.

Whelan, C.T. *The role of income, life-style deprivation and financial strain in mediating the impact of unemployment on psychological distress: evidence from the Republic of Ireland*. Unpublished mimeograph from The Economic and Social Research Institute, Dublin. c. 1991.

Whelan, C.T. The role of social support in mediating the psychological consequences of economic stress. *Sociology of Health and Illness* 15: 86–101. 1993.

White, M. *Against unemployment*. Policy Studies Institute, London. 1991.

Widdowson, E.M. Mental contentment and physical growth. *Lancet* June 16: 1316–18. 1951.

Wilkinson, R.G. *Poverty and progress: an ecological model of economic development*. Methuen, London. 1973.

Wilkinson, R.G. Income and mortality. In: *Class and health: research and longitudinal data*. Edited by R.G. Wilkinson. Tavistock, London. 1986.

Wilkinson, R.G. Class mortality differentials, income distribution and trends in poverty 1921–1981. *Journal of Social Policy* 18 (3): 307–35. 1989.

Wilkinson, R.G. Income distribution and mortality: a 'natural' experiment. *Sociology of Health and Illness* 12: 391–411. 1990.

Wilkinson, R.G. Income distribution and life expectancy. *British Medical Journal* 304: 165–8. 1992.

Wilkinson, R.G. The epidemiological transition: from material scarcity to social disadvantage? *Daedalus*. (Journal of The American Academy of Arts and Sciences). 123 (4): 61–77. 1994a.

Wilkinson, R.G. Health, redistribution and growth. In: *Paying for inequality: the economic cost of social injustice.* Edited by A. Glyn and D. Miliband. Rivers Oram Press, London. 1994b.

Wilkinson, R.G. *Unfair shares: the effects of widening income differentials on the welfare of the young.* Barnardos, Ilford. 1994c.

Wilkinson, R.G. A reply to Ken Judge: mistaken criticisms ignore overwhelming evidence. *British Medical Journal* 311: 1285–7. 1995.

Wilkinson, R.G. Health and comradeship: a hypothesis. In: *Environmental and non-environmental determinants of the East–West life expectancy gap in Europe.* Edited by C. Hertzman, S. Kelly and M. Bobak. Kluwer Academic, Amsterdam. 1996.

Wilson, S.H. and Walker, G.M. Unemployment and health: a review. *Public Health* 107: 153–62. 1993.

Winkelstein, M.L. and Feldman, H.L. Psychosocial predictors of consumption of sweets following smoking cessation. *Research in Nursing and Health* 16: 97–105. 1993.

Winter, J.M. *The Great War and the British people.* Macmillan, London. 1985.

Winter, J.M. Public health and the extension of life expectancy 1901–60. In: *The political economy of health and welfare.* Edited by M. Keynes. Cambridge University Press, Cambridge. 1988.

Wnuk-Lipinski, E. and Illsley, R. Introduction. *Social Science and Medicine* 31: 833–6. 1990.

Wolf, S. and Bruhn, J.G. *The power of clan; a 25-year prospective study of Roseto, Pennsylvania.* Transaction Publishers, New Brunswick, NJ. 1993.

Wolf, W. Verzerrungen durch Antwortausfalle in der Konsumerhebung 1984. *Statistische Nachrichten.* OSTAT, Vienna 43 (11): 861–7. 1988.

Woodburn, J. Egalitarian societies. *Man* 17: 431–51. 1982.

Woodroffe, C., Glickman, M., Barker, B. and Power, C. (eds) *Children, teenagers and health.* Open University Press, Milton Keynes. 1993.

World Bank, *The East Asian Miracle.* Oxford University Press, Oxford. 1993.

Name index

Subject index